# PRACTICE CALCULATIONS
## FOR THE
# NURSING STUDENT

Solving Fundamental, IV, and Pediatric Dosage
Calculations Accurately and with Confidence

**Written by**
**Diane L. Rhodes, MSN, APN, CHPN**

This book is dedicated to my students from whom I have learned so much.

Published 2019

Printed in the United States of America
Print ISBN: 978-1-7338384-8-1

Canoe Tree Press
4697 Main Street
Manchester, VT 05255

www.CanoeTreePress.com

# ABOUT THIS BOOK – A NOTE FROM THE AUTHOR

In 2005, I created a course for incoming nursing students because of perceived difficulties new nursing students had with writing care plans and with performing needed dosage calculations at different levels during nursing school. The course was designed to introduce students to dosage calculations *before the students ever take their first nursing class*, to introduce students to the needed concepts before they are needed for specific classes (fundamentals, med/surg, and pediatrics). This was intended to both increase student competency in doing dosage calculations, and to increase their confidence in their own ability to do these calculations correctly.

After taking the 13-day course, students repeatedly asked if there were additional practice problems they could do. Students who had not taken the course were asking the same question: where can we find additional problems to practice dosage calculations in the specific area of our next course? They told me on-line resources were limited, and not always easy to find.

In response, I created this book, which contains an introduction to how to do various problems at the three levels (fundamentals, IV math, and pediatric math), followed by 150 problems in each of the three areas. Thus, for example, in dealing with IV math, we look at time problems, 24-hour total parenteral intake problems, and reconstitution problems, before seeing 150 practice problems in IV math.

One of the greatest benefits of this book, according to student feedback, is the answer section. For each problem, not only is the answer to the problem given, *but also the setup of the problem to reach that answer.* Thus, if a student works a problem and gets the wrong answer, he or she can immediately see where they went wrong in the setup of the problem.

Because dosage calculations are so vital in nursing practice, and because nursing students are required to take dosage calculation exams numerous times during nursing school, this book was created. I hope it is helpful to students in giving them the ability to correctly calculate patient doses of medications both while in school and when they are in practice, and in allowing them to *know* they can do it right.

# TABLE OF CONTENTS

# BACKGROUND MATERIAL

# CONVERSIONS

| Metric | Household | Apothecary |
|---|---|---|
| 1000 mcg = 1 mg | | |
| 1000 mg = 1 g | | |
| 1000 g = 1 Kg | | |
| 1000 ml = 1 L | | |
| 1 ml | 15 gtt (drops) | |
| 60 mg | | 1 gr |
| 1 g (this one is rarely used) | | 15 gr |
| 15 g | 1 Tbsp (= 3 tsp) | |
| | 1 oz (= 2 Tbsp) | |
| 1 Kg | 2.2 lb | |
| 1 ml (=1 cc) | 15 gtt | |
| 5 ml* | 1 tsp | |
| 15 ml* | 1 Tbsp (= 3 tsp) | |
| 30 ml* | 1 oz (= 2 Tbsp) | |
| 480 ml* | 16 oz (= 1 pt = 2 c) | |
| 960 ml | 32 oz (= 1 qt = 2 pt) | |
| | | |
| 2.54 cm | 1 in | |
| 1 m | 39.4 in | |

And some basics:
1 ft = 12 in
1 lb = 16 oz

*Note that a few of the numbers are approximations for ease in calculation.

# ABBREVIATIONS

mcg = microgram

mg = milligram

g = gram

Kg = kilogram

Tbsp = tablespoon

tsp = teaspoon

oz = ounce

lb = pound

gr = grain

mEq = milliequivalent

ml = milliliter

L = liter

gtt = drops

pt = pint

c = cup

qt = quart

cm = centimeter

in = inch

m = meter

You may sometimes still see the following abbreviations, but they are no longer considered legitimate abbreviations as they are too easily misread (in a doctor's order, for example) as something else.

u or ut = unit

q = every or per, as in q 8 hr = every 8 hours

cc = cubic centimeter (= 1 ml)

# FORMS OF MEDICATIONS

PO = by mouth – tablets, capsules, caplets, liquid. Usually in mg or ml, sometimes gr, units, or gtt

IM = intramuscular – will be in ml

SQ = subcutaneous – will be in ml

intradermal – will be in ml

SL = sublingual – usually in mg or gtt

intrathecal = into the spinal canal – in ml

topical = onto the surface of the skin – will be in inches or mg

inhalants = inhaled into the nose or mouth – in mcg, mcg/spray, or mg, depending on form

ophthalmic = into the eye – will generally be in gtt

PR = rectally – will be in mg. Many PO meds can be given PR if necessary. (An example: the patient can no longer take tablets by mouth, as with decreased level of consciousness, and the medicine does not come in any other form.)

vaginal = into the vagina – will be in units or dispensers

IV = intravenously (into the vein) – will be in ml

# INTRODUCTION TO DIMENSIONAL ANALYSIS

First, a basic point: conversion factors can be written either way:

$$\frac{2.2\ \text{lb}}{1\ \text{Kg}} \quad \textbf{OR} \quad \frac{1\ \text{Kg}}{2.2\ \text{lb}}$$

Either way you write it, it says the same thing: that amount of lb and Kg are equal to one another, right? 1 Kg is always equal to 2.2 lb, regardless of how written. The numbers simply express a *relationship* between pounds and kilograms. In doing your calculations, you will write them whichever way is required by the problem.

Now, in doing dimensional analysis, there are some basic steps:

1.  Determine the form your answer is in. What does the question seek? Write that down as your starting point. Example: the question asks how many tablets you will give. You start by writing down tab =

2.  Determine the starting factor – a known quantity and unit. You should always start with what you are looking for in the answer. Example: you have 100 mg tabs available. Then

    $$\text{tab} = \frac{1\ \text{tab}}{100\ \text{mg}}$$

    Note that whatever you are looking for (tab) goes on *top* (numerator) after the equals sign, as shown here. Whatever is on the bottom (denominator) of the first factor (in this case, mg), must go on top (numerator) of the next factor. Let's say the doctor ordered 300 mg, so

    $$\text{tab} = \frac{1\ \text{tab}}{100\ \text{mg}} \times \frac{300\ \text{mg}}{\text{d.o.}} = 3 \text{ tabs. (d.o. = doctor's order)}$$

3.  Determine which conversion factors or other factors are needed, if any, OR write in any other information you need, such as the doctor's order.

4. Use simple math to solve. You multiply across the numerators, then multiply across the denominators, then divide your two numbers for the answer. Thus 1 x 300 = 300 (numerator), 100 (denominator), and 300/100 = 3 in our example.

You use dimensional analysis every day, without even realizing it. Here are several examples:

Example: How many feet in 9 yards?

$$\text{feet} = \frac{3 \text{ feet}}{1 \text{ yd}} \times 9 \text{ yards} = 27 \text{ ft}$$

Example: How many seconds in 5 minutes?

$$\text{seconds} = \frac{60 \text{ sec}}{1 \text{ min}} \times 5 \text{ min} = 300 \text{ sec}$$

Example: How many oz in 6 cups?

$$\text{ounces} = \frac{16 \text{ oz}}{2 \text{ c}} \times 6 \text{ cups} = 48 \text{ oz}$$

**NOTE that whatever you are looking for goes on top after the first = sign. In this case you are looking for ounces, so the ounces in your conversion factor must be on top: ounces = 16 OZ/2 c. Whatever is in the denominator of the numbers (in this case, cups) just to the right of the = sign (the first factor) will be in the numerator of the next factor, and so on. *This bottom/top arrangement allows you to cancel irrelevant information.* Thus, in the example we just looked at, cups would cancel out, leaving ounces, the desired answer. You must continue to add factors as necessary until every unit cancels out except the one(s) you are looking for in your answer. *In this way, you will <u>always</u> be able to tell when your setup is complete!***

Example: How many ml in 4 qt?

$$\text{ml} = \frac{960 \text{ ml}}{1 \text{ qt}} \times 4 \text{ qt} = 3840 \text{ ml}$$

Example: You received $325 in change, all quarters. How many did you get?

$$\text{qtrs.} = \frac{4 \text{ qtrs}}{1 \text{ dol}} \times 325 \text{ dol} = 1300 \text{ quarters}$$

Example: What is the weight in kg of a child weighing 40 lb?

$$kg = \frac{1\ kg}{2.2\ lb} \times 40\ lb = 18.18\ kg = 18.2\ kg$$

**So to repeat, then, the basic rule is: Always set up your first factor so unit in the numerator (top) of the first factor is what you are looking for in the answer.**

**Thereafter, the denominator in the first factor should be the numerator in the second factor; the denominator in that second factor should be the numerator in the third factor, and so on. In this way, all the units will cancel out, EXCEPT the one you need for your answer. When you can look at your work and see that this is true, you will know your setup is complete.**

### Two key points in doing nursing math:

1.  **There should never be more than a 10 percent difference between the ordered dose and the amount given. Whenever possible, you should give the exact dose ordered. Be sure your facility uses this 10% rule.**

2.  **Always ask: does my answer make sense? Very large amounts are suspect, e.g. 12 tabs PO, 15 ml IM. The numbers are illogical and unreasonable. Recheck your math and your setup. The most common error is a misplaced decimal.**

### Rounding:

For our purposes in this book, for Fundamentals math and Med/Surg I IV math, we will be consistent in our rounding: take the **answer** to two places and round to one (that is, to tenths). Thus, 18.18 kg becomes 18.2 kg, based on normal rounding rules. (If the number to be rounded is 5 or greater, round up, if less than 5, round down. Thus, the final 8 is greater than 5 in our 18.18, so causes the number to round to 18.2. Had the answer been 18.12, the answer would have rounded to 18.1, because the 2 is less than 5 in the basic rounding rule.)

For Pediatric math, we will take our answers to three places and round to two (in other words, round to hundredths in your answer). This is because even relatively small changes in amounts can make a big difference to very small patients.

Notice we are taking the **answer** to two or three places and then rounding. Usually, if you have a decimal in your problem, *do not round* until you get to the answer.

# RECONSTITUTION PROBLEMS

In addition to the basics already covered, we need to look at reconstitution.

At times, medications are reconstituted for use with a patient. The medicine may come as a powder or as a liquid available for reconstitution.

If it is in the form of a powder, the vial will state how much of the medication is inside, given as g or mg. Package directions will tell you how much liquid to add to produce the reconstituted medication. When you add this liquid, you need to realize *the powder does not change the total volume of fluid in the vial.* Thus, if you have 1 g powdered medicine in the vial and add 20 ml of fluid, your concentration is now 1g/20 ml (read the slash as "per"). If your problem states you have a 10 ml vial containing 1 g powdered medicine and add 8 ml of fluid, the available concentration of the vial's contents is now 1 g/8 ml. The vial size is irrelevant.

Let's look at that a little more. Note that a vial size may or may not be relevant. If your problem tells you that you have a 10 ml vial containing 50 mg/ml, the concentration is 50 mg/ml, and we don't care about the size of the vial. However, if instead the problem tells you that you have a 10 ml vial containing 500 mg, you have no concentration given, and the vial size becomes part of the concentration: 500 mg/10 ml. **This is the only time the vial size will become part of your calculations.**

If your medication is in the form of a liquid, the vial will again state how much of the medication is inside. Package directions will tell you how much fluid to add this medication to for a given dilution. At this time, you will add the fluid in the vial to the fluid which you are diluting, and then determine your final concentration. Thus, if you have 500 mg in 2 ml of fluid to start with, and add it to 50 ml of fluid, the concentration of your medication is now 500 mg/52 ml (that is, 500mg/50 ml + 2 ml).

On the other hand, if you have 500 mg/2 ml and your problem tells you to dilute it with 20 ml of sterile water, your available concentration is now 500 mg/22 ml.

Notice the difference in the situation in those last two paragraphs. In the first case, you have added your available concentration to a bag of fluid (the 50 ml in our example). In the second case, you are actually changing the concentration from 500 mg/2 ml, to 500 mg/22 ml.

In working many problems involving reconstitution, once you have determined the concentration of the medication as indicated above, **there are only two pieces of information needed** to determine how much to give your patient: the concentration of the available medication, and the doctor's order. There may be numerous other numbers in the problem, but they can usually be ignored. So how do you determine what the concentration is? It will always be an amount of medicine in an amount of fluid. For example, 500 mg/10 ml (read this as 500 mg per 10 ml).

In working problems involving reconstitution of a powdered medication, you may have a question asking how much fluid you would need to add to create a desired concentration. In this case, **you again need only two pieces of information**: the desired concentration and the amount of medication you have. Your answer will be in ml: how much <u>fluid</u> will you need? Then if you have a doctor's order regarding the dose he wants the patient to get, you follow the usual rule: use the concentration of available medication (which you just created), and the doctor's order. See example 3 on the next page.

Let's look at some examples:

## Example 1

You have available a vial of medication 25,000 mg in 2 ml NS. You are to add it to a 250 ml bag of NS, and then administer it at the rate of 900 mg an hour. How many ml will you give per hour?

What is the concentration in this problem? 25,000 mg in 2 ml. What is the doctor's order? 900 mg per hour.

ml = 252 ml/25,000 mg x 900 mg = 9.1 ml

## Example 2

The medication ordered comes in a powdered form with 20 mg in a large vial. You are to add 30 ml NS, and then give a 12 mg PO dose of the medication. How many ml will you give?

What is the concentration in this problem? 20 mg in 30 ml. What is the doctor's order? 12 mg.

ml = 30 ml/20 mg x 12 mg = 18 ml

## Example 3

A medication is available as a powder 250 mg per vial. You are to add enough fluid to create a 25 mg/ml strength, and then you are to give 15 mg of the reconstituted medication. What is the concentration to be created? 25 mg/ml. Doctor's order? 15 mg.

a.  How much fluid should you add to create the desired strength? Here we need first to see how much fluid we will need to add to the 250 mg vial to create the desired strength of 25 mg/ml. You do that this way:
ml = 1 ml/25 mg x 250 mg = 10 ml (conc we want x amt of med we have)

b.  How many ml should you give to follow the doctor's order? Now we take the medication in the concentration we have created, and follow the doctor's order.
ml = 1 ml/25 mg x 15 mg = 0.6 ml

## Example 4

The medication comes in 10 ml vials with a concentration of 100 mg/10 ml. (Note you have a concentration given, so the vial size is irrelevant.) The doctor's order is to dilute 50 mg of the medication in a 100 ml bag of IV fluid. How much medication should be added to the bag to meet the doctor's order?

What is the concentration? 100 mg/10 ml. What is the doctor's order? 50 mg. *Note that the bag size does* not *enter your calculations; you will simply add the amount you calculate* to *that bag size.*

ml = 10 ml/100 mg x 50 mg = 5 ml

So you will add 5 ml of medication to the 100 ml bag, which will now contain 105 ml.

This will affect the calculation of flow rates when we get to IV math, but we will go no further in this section.

# TUBE FEEDING PROBLEMS

You may be asked to calculate time for a tube feeding problem. For example, the patient has tube feeding at X ml/hr; at what time will his 500 ml bag be empty. Let's look at that one first.

Your patient is to receive 500 ml of fluid through his feeding tube, at 40 ml/hr. If you hang the bag at 0900, at what time will it be empty?

Here you need to know how many hours it will take to empty, so you are looking for hours.

$$Hr = \frac{1\ hour}{40\ ml} \times 500\ ml = 12.5 \text{ hours so if hung at 0900, complete at } \textbf{2130}$$

To write this out in words: we are looking for hours, so hour must go on top after the = sign. We know that in every hour, 40 ml runs into the patient, and there are 500 ml total to go in. Then we just do the math.

Let's look at another type of tube feeding problem:

You are to give your patient 470 ml of feeding. You start at 0900 at 20 ml an hour, and increase the rate by 10 ml every two hours until you reach 80 ml an hour. When will the bag be empty?

|  |  |  |
|---|---|---|
|  | 470 ml | to start |
| 0900 – 1100 20 ml/hr x 2 hours | – 40 ml | |
|  | 430 ml | remaining |
| 1100 – 1300 30 ml/hr x 2 hours | – 60 ml | |
|  | 370 ml | remaining |
| 1300 – 1500 40 ml/hr x 2 hours | – 80 ml | |
|  | 290 ml | remaining |
| 1500 – 1700 50 ml/hr x 2 hours | – 100 ml | |
|  | 190 ml | remaining |
| 1700 – 1900 60 ml/hr x 2 hours | – 120 ml | |
|  | 70 ml | remaining |
| 1900 – 2000 70 ml/hr x 1 hour | – 70 ml | |
|  | 0 ml | |

So **the bag will be empty at 2000**.

One more version of the same kind of problem. What if the question in the previous problem, rather than when the bag would be empty, had been "at what time would you set the feeding pump at 80 ml an hour?"

Well, you know that at 1900 you would set the pump at 70 ml/hr, for two hours, so **you would not have set it for 80 ml/hr until 2100.** (For the example shown, that was irrelevant, as the bag was empty at 2000.) Be careful to answer what was actually asked in these questions. It may ask when the bag may be empty, or when will you need to hang a new bag, or at what time the flow will reach a certain rate.

OK, we've covered the basics. Let's take a look at Fundamentals math.

One point should be made here: the problem may tell you what the answer's units will be. For example, it may ask, "How many tablets will you give?" Then you know the answer will be in tablets. However, what if it just asks, "How much will you give?" *You can only give the medicine in the form in which it comes. Thus, if it comes in a liquid form, you will be looking for ml.*

# FUNDAMENTAL NURSING DOSAGE CALCULATIONS

# FUNDAMENTAL DOSAGE CALCULATIONS

**Playing with conversions:**

1.      90 ml = _____ Tbsp = _____ tsp

2.      720 ml = _____ pints = _____ cups = _____ oz.

3.      How many drops in one cup?

4.      How many tsp in 1 pt?

5.    In lb, how much does a 45 Kg patient weigh?

6.    a.    Your patient weighed 54 Kg and was told to lose 10% of his body weight. He did so. How much did he lose, in lb?

      b.    Your patient weighed 300 lb and was told to lose 10% of his body weight. He did so. How much does he weigh now, in Kg?

7.    150 mg = _____ gr

8.    3.5 pt = _____ ml

9.    3000 mcg = _____ mg = _____ g

10.    14 oz = _____ ml

**And now, some regular fundamentals math problems:**

11.    Order: 60 mg codeine PO
       Available: codeine gr ½ per tab
       How many tabs should you give?

12.    Order: Reglan 20 mg
        Available: Reglan 10 mg/ml
       How many ml should you give?

13.    Order: Nembutal gr v PO [grains may be given in Roman numerals]
       Available: Nembutal 100 mg capsules
       How many caps will you give?

14. Order: oxycodone 50 mg PO
    Available: oxycodone oral solution 20 mg/ml
    How much will you give?

15. Order: ethambutol 15 mg/kg/24 hours PO to an adult
    weighing 176 lb.
    Label: ethambutol 400 mg/tab
    How many tabs should you give?

16. Doctor's order: tetracycline 350 mg PO
    Available: tetracycline suspension 125 mg/ml
    How much will you give?

17. Order: levothyroxine 0.075 mg PO daily
    Available: levothyroxine 50 mcg/tab
    How many tabs will you give?

18. The medication comes as 500 mg in a powdered form, to which you are to add 75 ml of sterile water. The doctor's order is for 400 mg one-time PO dose. How much will you give?

19. Phenergan 75 mg PO ordered
    Phenergan syrup 25 mg/5 ml available
    How many tsp should you give? (Note: here you must start with a conversion factor.)

20. Order: Nembutal sodium gr 1.5 PO
    Label: Nembutal sodium 100 mg/cap
    How many caps should you give?

**Remember: up to a 10% difference between what is ordered and what is given is still OK.**

21.   Order: PCN 800,000 units IM
      Available: PCN 1,000,000 units per ml
      How much will you give the patient?

**Note: If your answer is a decimal less than 1, you must put a zero before the decimal.**

22.   Order: 30 mg Nitro-Dur transdermally, change every 6 hours.
      Available: 1 in = 15 mg (Note: Nitro-Dur is a paste)

      a.    How much will you give per dose?

      b.    How much will you give per day?

23.   Order: dilute the medication with 80 ml of NS, and give a 20 mg IV dose.
      Available: vial of medication containing 200 mg in 2 ml, which you are to dilute.
      How much will you give?

24.   Lovenox 1 mg/kg SQ has been ordered. It is available in a preloaded syringe of 80
      mg/0.8 ml. Your patient weighs 165 lb. How many mg will you give? How many ml?

25. A COPD patient comes in in respiratory distress, and the ER physician orders Solumedrol 60 mg IV push. The drug is available as 125 mg in 2 ml. How many ml will you give?

26. Order: Clindamycin 225 mg IM every 6 hr for 7 days
Available: Clindamycin 75 mg/ml in a 5 ml vial

    a. How much will you give with each dose?

    b. What is the total dosage the doctor has ordered, in mg?

27. Valproic acid is ordered 15 mg/kg/day. It is available as 250 mg caps. Your patient weighs 73 pounds. How much will he get per day in mg? How many capsules?

28. The patient is to receive 240 ml via feeding tube. You start the feeding at 0700 at 20 ml/hr, and have instructions to increase the rate every hour, by 10 ml/hr to a maximum of 50 ml/hr. At what time will the bag be empty?

29. The medication is a powder, 500 mg per vial. You are to add enough fluid to create a 40 mg/ml concentration. How much fluid will you add?

30. Your patient weighs 44 pounds. You are to give 0.5 mg/kg of a medication, per dose. The medication comes in a concentration of 5 mg/ml. How much will you give?

31. The doctor has ordered iii grains of phenobarbital every eight hours. The medication comes in 2 ml vials containing 65 mg/ml. How much will you give per dose?

32. The oral solution ordered is available 2 g in 100 ml. The doctor's order is for 300 mg. How much will you give in ml?

33. The doctor's order reads digoxin 375 mcg daily. The tablets available are 0.125 mg. How many tablets should you give?

34. Your patient is to get 12 mEq of potassium every 6 hours. The potassium available comes 40 mEq per packet, to be dissolved in 30 ml of juice. How much should you give per dose?

35. The order is for 8 mg of methadone. Methadone is available in a 10 ml vial, with a concentration of 5 mg/ml. How much will you give?

36. Ordered: 1/120 gr digoxin (Change fractions to decimals; don't round till the answer)
    Available: 0.25 mg tablets
    How many tablets will you give?

37. Your patient is to get 800,000 units of penicillin. The penicillin available comes 200,000 units/ml in a 10 ml vial. How much will you give?

38. Aspirin is available in 10 gr tablets. The doctor's order is for 1200 mg every four hours. How many tabs will you give per dose?

39. An antibiotic has been ordered, 0.2 g four times daily. The available medication is 100 mg per capsule. How many capsules will you give per day?

40. Robinul comes in a 5 ml vial containing 0.2 mg/ml. The doctor has ordered 0.4 mg every four hours as needed for congestion. Your patient requires four doses in a 24-hour period. How much was that in ml?

41. Tube feeding is to give 400 ml starting at 0700. You are to start it at 20 ml/hr, increasing by 20 ml/hr every 2 hours to a maximum of 80 ml/hr. (a) At what time would that rate be reached? (b) When would the bag be empty?

42. The order is for phenobarbital 70 mg twice a day; available is phenobarbital 65 mg/1 ml. How much will you give per dose? Per day?

43. You are to give 1800 units of a medication. The available dose strength is 1000 units per 1.5 ml. How much will you give?

44. The doctor's order is for 5 mg of Lasix. The pharmacy has it available in a 2 ml vial, 10 mg per ml. How much should you give?

45. Order: 260 mcg Robinul. Available: Robinul 0.2 mg/ml in a 10 ml vial. Your patient should receive how much?

46. The available medication comes 1200 mg in a 2.5 ml vial. The doctor has ordered 800 mg. Calculate the patient's dose.

47. Order: 170 mg of a medication. It is available in a liquid form, 100 mg/ml. Dose:

48. A medication which comes 1.5 mg in 2 ml is to be used to prepare a 0.75 mg dosage for your patient. How much fluid will be required in order to accurately mix the correct dose?

49. You are to add 600 mg of a medication to an IV bag (although normally the pharmacy does this). The solution available to use comes 500 mg in 10 ml. How much will you add?

50. You are to prepare a 0.6 g dose from a 300 mg per 2 ml solution. How much will you need?

51. You are to add enough fluid to a 75 mg vial to create a 30mg/ml concentration, then give a 22 mg dose. How much fluid should you add, and how much (in ml) will you give?

52. The order is for 2 tsp of cough syrup every 4 hours. Available: 10 mg/ml

    a.   How many gtt will the patient get per dose?

    b.   How many mg will the patient get per dose?

53. The order is for Equamil 0.2 g by mouth every 4 hours.
    Available: Equamil 400 mg per tab

    a.   How many mg would you give per dose?

    b.   How many tabs would this be?

c.   How many tabs would you give in 48 hours?

54.   Order: 0.6 g PO every 6 hours
      Available: 200 mg/5 ml
      Give: _____ ml in 24 hours

55.   You have reconstituted a medicine, creating a strength of 100 mg/ml.
      The order is to give 0.3 g every 8 hours. Total dose in 3 days?
      (Remember, you can only give medicine in the form it comes in, which here is a liquid,
      so you are looking for ml.)

56.   At 0800 you begin a G-tube feeding of 930 ml, starting at 30 ml/hr. The MD's orders
      say to increase the rate hourly by 10 ml/hr to a maximum of 80 ml/hr.

      a.   At what time will the rate reach 80 ml/hr?

      b.   At what time will the bag be empty?

57. The patient is to get 30 mg/Kg/day of a medication in three divided doses. He weighs 187 lb. The medication is available 100 mg/ml.

    a.    mg per dose?

    b.    ml per day?

58. Order: 1.5 mg/Kg/day for a patient who weighs 92.6 Kg
Available: 125 mg/ml

    a.    How many ml/day will the patient receive?

    b.    How many mg will he receive in 48 hours?

59. Order: gr iii phenobarbital every 6 hours prn agitation
Available: 60 mg tablets
How many tablets will you give per dose?

60. The patient is to receive 0.2 units/Kg of insulin.
    The patient weighs 320 lb. The insulin is available 100 units/ml.

    a. How many units will the patient receive? (Remember, for units you must round to the nearest whole number.)

    b. How many ml will that be? (Round to nearest tenth.)

61. The doctor has ordered 60 mg of Phenergan. It is available 20 mg/5 ml.
    How many tsp should you give?

62. Clindamycin has been ordered 250 mg IM every 6 hours for 7 days.
    It is available 50 mg/ml in a 5 ml vial.
    How much will you need (in mg) for the 7-day supply?
    How many vials would that be?

63. You are to add 700 mg of a medication to an IV bag.
    The solution available comes 250 mg in 5 ml. How much will you add?

64. The order is for Procan 500 mg loading dose (a large initial dose, intended to begin setting up a given level in the patient's bloodstream), followed by 250 mg every 3 hours. Available: Procan 100 mg tabs.

    a.    How many tabs will you give as a loading dose?

    b.    How many tabs will you give for each dose after the loading dose?

    c.    After the loading dose is given, how many additional tabs will you need for the next 24 hours?

65. The order is for metronidazole 3 g per day in 4 equal divided doses. The medicine is available as 500 mg tabs. How many tabs will you give with each dose?

66. Glycopyrrolate 0.1 mg is ordered. Glycopyrrolate is available in 10 ml vials with a concentration of 0.2 mg/ml. How many ml will you give your patient?

67. You are to give your patient 750 mg of a medication available 0.3 g in 1 ml. How much will you give?

68. Cefotaxime comes in 50 ml vials with a concentration of 300 mg/ml. The doctor's order is for 60 mg/Kg/dose, with one dose every 6 hours. The patient weighs 30 Kg.

   a. How much will you give per dose?

   b. How much will you give per day?

69. You are to reconstitute a vial of 50,000 units of urokinase to a concentration of 2000 units per ml. How much diluent will you use?

70. Available scored tablets come in three sizes: 10, 20, and 40 gr. The doctor has ordered 1200 mg of the medication. How many tablets would you give of each tablet size to follow the doctor's order? (Solve the problems using the fewest number of tablets possible, and without cutting any tablets.)

   a. 10 gr

b. 20 gr

c. 40 gr

71. Order: Nembutal gr iii PO
Available: Nembutal 90 mg capsules
How many capsules will you give?

72. The doctor has ordered gr ii of phenobarbital for the agitated patient.
The medication is available in 2 ml vials containing 130 mg/ml of phenobarbital.
How much will you give your patient?

73. The order is for 1/120 gr of a medication which is available in 0.25, 0.5, and 1 mg tablets.
Which will you give? (Give fewest tabs possible.)

74. Your patient weighs 66 pounds. You are to give 0.5 mg/Kg of a medication per dose, twice a day. The medication comes in a concentration of 5 mg/ml. How much will you give per day?

75. Your patient is to get 8 mEq of potassium every 4 hours.
The potassium available comes 40 mEq per packet, to be dissolved in 30 ml of juice.
How much should you give per dose?

76. An antibiotic has been ordered 0.4 g six times daily. Available are 200 mg capsules of the antibiotic. How many capsules will you give per day?

77. The doctor has ordered 1/120 gr digoxin.
The pharmacy has 0.25 mg tablets.
How many tablets should you give to obey the MD's order?

78. The doctor has ordered cefoxitin 75 mg/Kg/day, in 6 equal doses (that is, a dose every 4 hours). The medicine is available 1.5 g in 100 ml of D5W. The patient weighs 88 pounds.

    a.   How much is the patient receiving per day, in mg?

    b.   How much should you give per dose in ml?

79. Flecainide, an antiarrhythmic, is available in 50, 100, and 150 mg scored tablets. Which tablets will you choose for a 500 mg daily dose, and how many tablets will you give? (The rules: use the fewest number of tabs possible. Do not cut tabs if you can give the dose without doing so. You can give more than one size tab in a single dose.)

80. The doctor orders 35 mEq of potassium for your hypokalemic patient. The medication comes in 10 or 20 mEq capsules, so you can't use either of those, since capsules can't be split. An oral solution with 20 mEq in 15 ml is available. How much will you give? (Round to the nearest 100th.)

81. The MD has ordered a medication with dose based on the size of the patient. The patient is to get 5 mg/Kg of the medication. The patient weighs 209 pounds.

   a.   How many mg of medicine will he receive?

   b.   If the medication is available 50 mg/ml, how many ml should you give the patient?

82. PCN G comes in a vial containing 10,000,000 units.
    You are to reconstitute it to a concentration of 400,000 units/ml.
    How much diluent must you add to the vial?

83. The medication prescribed is available 50 mg in 200 ml.
    The doctor has ordered 30 mg per day in three divided doses.
    How much should you give per dose?

84. The order is for levofloxacin by mouth, with an initial (first) order of 400 mg, followed by 250 mg three times daily thereafter. Only 100 mg tablets are available.

   a.   How many tablets will be in the initial dose?

   b.   How many tablets will be in each subsequent dose?

85. The doctor has ordered a loading dose of 450 mg of a medication, followed by a 300 mg dose every 6 hours for one week. The medication comes in 150 mg tablets. Not counting the loading dose (so the clock starts six hours after the loading dose), how many tablets will be needed for one week?

86. The patient is having chest pain, so the doctor orders nitroglycerin paste 30 mg every 6 hours. The medication comes as a paste in small packets containing 15 mg = 1 inch. How many packets will be required for one day?

87. The medication is to be given at 3 mg/Kg/dose to a patient weighing 242 pounds. The medication is available 100 mg/ml. How much will you give per dose, in ml?

88. The patient is to be fed via G tube. The MD orders a 300 ml initial feeding to test the patient's tolerance, starting at 30 ml/hr and increasing by 10 ml/hr every 2 hours to a maximum of 60 ml/hr. At what time will you set the rate at 60 ml/hr, assuming you start the feeding at 1800?

89. The doctor has ordered 4 grains per day of a medication which is available only in 30 mg tablets. The ordered reads "4 gr in 4 divided doses." How many tablets will the patient receive per dose?

90. Your patient is to receive 650 ml of fluid through a G tube. You start the feeding at 20 ml/hr at 0700, and orders are to increase it by 20 ml/hr every two hours to a maximum of 80 ml/hr. At what time will the bag be empty?

91. Order: 1/150 gr of a medication
    Available: 0.2 mg tablets
    How many tablets will you give per dose?

92. Your patient is to receive 50 mg of a medication which comes 5 mg/ml. How many tsp will she get?

93. The medication is available 250 mg in 2 ml NS. The doctor has ordered 700 mg. How much will the patient receive?

94. The patient's order is for 15 mcg per Kg. The medication is available 1 mg/ml. How much will the patient receive if he weighs 115 Kg?

95. You are to reconstitute a powdered medication which comes 500 mg in a 10 ml vial.
    You add 8 ml of sterile water to the vial.
    The doctor's order is for 275 mg.
    How much will that be in ml?

96. The doctor has ordered v grains of a medication which is available only in 300 mg tablets. How many tablets will you give?

97. The medication was ordered as an oral solution containing 10 mg/ml.
    The doctor has ordered a 250 mg dose every 6 hours.
    How much will the patient receive in one day?

98. The doctor has ordered the patient to receive feedings through a G tube. He has ordered the feedings be started at 20 ml/hr, then increased by 20 ml/hr every two hours until the patient is receiving 100 ml/hr.
You hang a 500 ml bag at 0900. At what time will the bag be empty?

99. You are to dilute 2 g of a powdered medication in a vial to create a concentration of 250 mg/ml. How much diluent should you add?

100. In the previous question, if the doctor has ordered a 50 mg dose of the medication, how much would you give?

101. Your 110 lb patient has medication ordered at 60 mg/Kg per day, in four divided doses. The tablets available are 50 mg, 100 mg, 250 mg, and 500 mg. You are to give the fewest number of tablets possible (do NOT cut tablets if possible), and can use more than one tablet size to make up the dose. Which tablet(s) should be given per dose?

102. The medication is available 600 mg in a vial.
You must add enough diluent to create a strength of 75 mg per ml.
How much should you add to the vial?

103. The doctor has ordered a 250 mg dose every 8 hours for 7 days.
The medication comes in 100 mg and 50 mg tablets.
How many of each would you need to order for a 7-day supply?

104. Penicillin 600,000 units IM is ordered for your patient.
PCN is available in a vial containing one million units per ml.
How much has the doctor ordered you to give?

105. The medication is available 500 mg in 2 ml.
     You are to dilute this with 50 ml of NS, then give a 60 mg dose every 6 hours.
     How much will you give the patient per dose?

106. The doctor has ordered iii grains of a medication which is available 130 mg/ml.
     How much will you give?

107. A powdered medication is available 300 mg in a vial.
     You must add enough diluent to create a concentration of 50 mg/ml.
     How much diluent will you add?

108. How much of the newly reconstituted medication in the previous problem would you
     draw up to give a 75 mg dose?

109. Again based on the medication in problem 107, how much of the medication will be present in 3.5 ml?

110. The doctor has ordered 500 mcg of a medication, which is available at your facility only as 0.125 mg tablets. How many tablets will you need to give?

111. The patient is to get 1 g per day of a medication, in four divided doses.
The medication is available in 125 mg capsules.
How many capsules will your patient receive per dose?

112. The doctor has ordered 12 mg/Kg every 6 hours for your 110 pound patient.
Tablets available are 150 mg.
How many tablets will your patient receive in one day?

113.  The medication is available in 15 mg, 30 mg, 60 mg, and 100 mg tablets. It is also available in a solution with a concentration of 50 mg/ml.
Your patient, who weighs 35 Kg, has the medication ordered at 4 mg/Kg.
Would you give tablets or the solution, and why?

114.  For the previous problem, calculate how much of the available medication you would give.

115.  The patient has an oral, liquid form of morphine ordered hourly prn (as needed) for pain. The medication is available 20 mg/ml. The doctor's order reads 5 mg for mild pain, 10 mg for moderate pain, and 20 mg for severe pain. During your shift, you dose the patient twice for mild pain, four times for moderate pain, and twice for severe pain. How many ml of the medication did you give on your shift?

116.  An oral solution is available 5 g in 100 ml. The doctor has ordered 250 mg. How much will you give?

117. The order is for 6 mg of a medication which comes 4 mg/ml in a 10 ml vial. How much will you give your patient?

118. The ordered potassium comes only in a powdered form with 20 mEq in each small packet, which must be dissolved in 15 ml of fluid.
The patient is to get 30 mEq of potassium every 8 hours.
How many ml will he get per day?

119. You are to add 800 mg of a medication to an IV bag, using a reconstituted solution with a concentration of 500 mg in 8 ml. How much will you add?

120. The medication comes as a 100 mg powder.
You are to add enough diluent to create a concentration of 25 mg/ml.
How much will you add?

121. You are to give 1 g of a medication in four divided doses.
How much will you give per dose?

122. The doctor has ordered 2 g daily in four divided doses. 250 mg tablets are available.
How many tablets would you need for a 10-day supply?

123. The ordered medication is available in a concentration of 0.03 mg/ml.
The doctor has ordered 90 mcg. How much will you give (in ml)?

124. The general rule is to give the fewest number of tablets needed to provide the ordered dose, and to avoid cutting tablets if possible.
The patient has an order for ¾ gr of medication.
The medication is available in 15, 30, and 60 mg scored tablets.
How will you give the dose? (Remember, you can use more than one size tablet to create the ordered dose.)

125. The patient is to receive continuous feeding through his G tube, starting with a 300 ml bag. He is to start at 30 ml/hr, and you are to increase the rate by 10 ml/hr, checking residual every two hours and stopping the feeding for one hour if there is an hour's worth or more of feeding (at the current rate) in the residual. Maximum rate per the doctor's order is to be 60 ml/hr. If you start the feeding at 1000, at what time will you need to hang a new bag, assuming no excessive residual?

126. The doctor has ordered 600,000 units of PCN every 6 hours for the patient. The PCN comes in a vial with a concentration of 2 million units in 5 ml. How much will the patient receive per day?

127. Order: 1/6 gr
Available: Elixir with a concentration of 10 mg/2 ml.
How much has been ordered?

128. The ordered sliding scale is:

| | |
|---|---|
| 0 – 150 | 0 units of regular insulin |
| 150 – 249 | 3 units |
| 250 – 349 | 5 units |
| 350 – 400 | 8 units |
| Over 400 | 10 units and call the doctor |

You check your patient's blood sugar, and it is 323. The insulin comes in a concentration of 50 units per ml. Following the sliding scale, how much will you give your patient?

129. The patient is to receive 1.5 g of medication daily, in six divided doses.
The medication comes 5 g in a 250 ml bag of IV fluids.
How much will the patient receive per dose?

130. The doctor has ordered 750 mg of a medication in a 100 ml IV bag which will be given over a one hour period once daily. You are to reconstitute the medication to create a concentration of 150 mg/ml before adding it to the bag. How much diluent will you use?

131. Your patient is to receive a medication at 12 mg/Kg per day, with a dose given every 8 hours. Your patient weighs 99 pounds. How much will she get per dose?

132. Order: 30 mg
Available: 500 mcg/ml
How much will you give?

133. Order: 300 mg
Available: 10 ml vial with 2 g of medication in it
How much will you give?

134. You have reconstituted a powdered medication and now have a 10 ml vial containing 3 g of medication. The doctor wants 750 mg in a 100 ml bag of IV solution.
How much of your reconstituted medication should you add to the bag?

135. You have received an order for your patient of 1/120 gr of a medication.
How much is that, in mg?

136. A powdered medication comes 400 mg in a vial.
You are to add enough of a diluent to the vial to create a 125 mg/ml concentration.
How much diluent will you add?

137. The doctor has ordered 60 mg of a medication which is available 3 mg/ml.
How many tsp will the patient receive?

138. The patient is to receive 25 mg/Kg per day in four divided doses.
How much will the patient receive per dose? (The patient weighs 58 pounds.)

139. The order is for 1.5 g of medication to be given daily, divided into one dose every four hours. How much should be given per dose?

140. You are to give a tube feeding at 0900, starting at 20 ml/hr and increasing the rate every 2 hours by 10 ml/hr. At what time will you reach the ordered rate of 70 ml/hr?

141. Order: 1/6 gr of a medication
Available: medication containing 1/120 gr per ml
How many ml has the doctor ordered?

142. Your patient is to get Roxanol, a liquid form of morphine, prn for pain.
The order reads: 5 mg for mild pain (1-3 on 10-point scale), 10 mg for moderate pain (4-7 on the scale), 20 mg for severe pain (8-10 on the scale), hourly as needed. During your shift, you give 4 doses for mild pain, 2 for moderate pain, and 4 for severe pain.
The medication is available 20 mg/ml. How much did you give, in ml, during your shift?

143. Order: 300 mg of a medication
Available: Elixir 40 mg/ml
How much will you give?

144. The doctor has ordered 3 grains of phenobarbital for a patient's agitation.
The medication is available in a liquid form of 65 mg/ml.
How much will you give?

145. Your 206.8 pound patient is to receive a medication ordered at 12 mg/Kg/24 hours, in three divided doses. The medication comes as 375 mg tablets. How many tablets will he get per dose?

146. The medication comes in the form of 0.5 g powder in a 10 ml vial.
You are to create a concentration of 250 mg/ml.
How much diluent must you add?

147. Order: 750 mg of a medication
Available: 1 g in a 5 ml vial
How much will you give?

148. The patient is to receive a tube feeding of 630 ml of Jevity. Because she has not
previously had tube feedings, the doctor is not sure what rate she will tolerate.
He therefore orders the feeding to begin at 20 ml/hr, increasing by 10 ml/hr every
hour, to a maximum of 80 ml/hr. You start the feeding at 0800. At what time will the
bag be empty?

149. The doctor has ordered 500 mg of a medication four times daily.
The medication comes from the pharmacy in the form of 250 mg tablets.
How many tablets will be needed for a three-day supply?

150. The order is for 1 unit/Kg of insulin for your 200-pound patient.
How many units will the patient receive?
(Remember, the answer for insulin must be rounded to the nearest whole number.)

# IV DOSAGE CALCULATIONS

# MED/SURG IV MATH

## DEFINITIONS

**Flow rate** = infusion rate = hourly rate. All of these indicate a pump is in use. The pump can "read" <u>only</u> ml/hr, so if any of these terms are used to describe what you are looking for, your answer should be in **ml/hr**. Example: "At what rate will this medication infuse?" You are looking for an infusion rate, so your answer will be in ml/hr. (Note: this is ml per *hour*. Ml/0.5 hour, ml/0.75 hr, ml/1.5 hr are *not* flow rates.)

**Drip rate** – this is another way of determining how fast a medication is going in (infusing). If asked for a drip rate, your answer should always be in **gtt/min**. (Gtt is drops.) The answer must always be a whole number, as there is no way to accurately measure a partial drop.

**Drop factor** is simply the size of the tubing. It is literally the number of drops it takes to make up one ml, using that particular tubing. It is therefore always given as **gtt/ml**. Watch your step – that's drops per **ml**, <u>not</u> per minute. Don't confuse this with drip rate.

## TWO KEY FORMULAS

DRIP RATE = DROP FACTOR X FLOW RATE

(FLOW RATE = CONCENTRATION X DOCTOR'S ORDER.)

This second formula is true **ONLY** when the doctor's order for infusion is given in something other than ml/hr, such as mg/hr or mEq/hr.

## A FURTHER LOOK AT TUBING SIZE (drop factor)

There are two types of tubing: macro and micro.

**MICRO** tubing is used primarily with pediatric and geriatric patients. It is used when the flow rate (ml/hr) is **less than 100**. (There are two exceptions to this: if you are giving blood, or if you are hanging a viscous (thick and sticky) fluid, you *must* use macro tubing, regardless of the flow rate.) Micro tubing comes in only one size: **60 gtt per ml**.

*Please note: Many facilities will choose to buy only one size tubing to save money, and this will be <u>macro</u> tubing, regardless of flow rate or patient size. Therefore, if you are doing drip rate problems in the clinical setting, you <u>can</u> and <u>must</u> use <u>only</u> the drop factor of the tubing available at your facility.*

Back to our tubing:

**MACRO** tubing is used only when the flow rate (ml/hr) is **100 or more**. (Many hospitals have *only* macro tubing, so you may have to use it even though the medication and rate really calls for micro tubing.) Macro tubing comes in three sizes: **10, 15, and 20 gtt per ml**. In solving problems on the test or in clinical, sometimes the drop factor will not be given/known, so you must decide if macro or micro tubing should be used (based on flow rate). If it is macro, you can use any of the three sizes of tubing, and (if your math is correct) your answer will be correct. Remember: If you are in the clinical setting, you <u>must</u> use the tubing size available at that facility in doing your calculations.


## ANOTHER CONSIDERATION

If a problem involves heparin or insulin, something that comes in units, be very careful to check what response the question is asking for in your answer, because it may be units or ml. **If a question is asking about dosage or dosage per hour**, the answer must be in the form (ml, mg, units, etc.) the medicine comes in. Thus, if a question about insulin asks for hourly dosage, your answer would be in units/hr.

### A couple of examples of IV math

1.  Patient has D5.45NS infusing at 150 ml/hr. What is the drip rate?

    Drip rate = drop factor x flow rate. 150 ml/hr is macro, so you can use 10, 15, or 20 gtt/ml for the drop factor. We'll use 10.

    gtt/min = 10 gtt/ml x 150 ml/60 min = 25 gtt/min

2.  A heparin drip is ordered to infuse at 900 units/hr. The IV solution is 25,000 units heparin in 250 ml D5W. What is the infusion rate?

Infusion rate = flow rate = concentration x doctor's order

ml/hr = 250 ml/25,000 units x 900 units/hr = 9 ml/hr

# TIME PROBLEMS

You will sometimes be asked to determine how long a fluid will take to infuse. If a question asks you, "How long," your answer can <u>only</u> be given in the form of time. After all, if you said you were going to the grocery, and someone said, "How long will you be gone?" you wouldn't answer, "Oh, about 125 ml/hr!"

Whether you initially determine your answer in hours or minutes will depend on what you have given in the problem.

## Hours

How long will it take a liter of NS to infuse at 75 ml/**hour**? You have hours in the problem, so let's find hours.

hr = 1 hr/75 ml x 1000 ml = 13.33 hours

What is this in hours and minutes? It is 13 hours plus 0.33 hour. One hour = 60 minutes, so it is 13 hours plus 0.33 hr x 60 min/hr = 20 minutes.

## Minutes

The doctor has ordered a 750 ml bolus dose of NS. Tubing size is 20 gtt/ml, and the drip rate is 30 gtt/**minute**. How long will it take to infuse? You have minutes in the problem, so let's start there.

min = 1 min/30 gtt x 20 gtt/ml x 750 ml = 500 min

Now turn this into hours and minutes. Eight hours = 480 minutes. 500 minutes - 480 minutes = 20 minutes, so the answer is 8 hours and 20 minutes.

# 24-HOUR TOTAL IV FLUIDS PROBLEMS

In these problems, you have a patient who is receiving multiple IV fluids. You need to determine how much fluid he is getting by IV in a 24-hour period, possibly because he is on fluid restriction.

Let's look at a problem: The patient is receiving lactated Ringers (LR) at 125 ml/hr. He also has three antibiotics ordered: Keflex 1 g in 100 ml twice daily (infused over 30 minutes), Cipro 500 mg in 50 ml three times daily (infused over 30 minutes), and Levaquin 2 g in 250 ml daily (infused over 1 hour). How much (in ml) is the patient receiving IV daily?

Start with the three secondary fluids, the antibiotics. To determine how much of each of them the patient is receiving per day, <u>all</u> that is needed is the volume of each per dose, and the number of doses per day. For this problem, then:

| | | | |
|---|---|---|---|
| Keflex | ml/day = 100 ml/dose | x 2 doses/day = | 200 ml |
| Cipro | ml/day = 50 ml/dose | x 3 doses/day = | 150 ml |
| Levaquin | ml/day = 250 ml/dose | x 1 dose /day = | 250 ml |
| Then add them together: | | TOTAL: | 600 ml |

The three secondary fluids total 600 ml in a day. *Note that time <u>does not</u> affect the volume of the secondary fluids in any way.* <u>Time</u> affects <u>only</u> the fluid that expresses itself in time, the primary fluid (the LR in our problem) that here runs at 125 ml <u>per hour</u>.

Now, an important thing to know is that the pump can run only one fluid at a time. Thus, when the antibiotics/secondary fluids run, the primary fluid (the LR) stops. So we cannot just say 125 ml/hr x 24 hours for the total LR the patient gets in 24 hours.

We have to look at the secondary fluids again. How long does it take for one dose of Keflex to run in? 30 minutes. How many doses a day? Two. So for one hour a day, Keflex is running in, and LR is not. We could express it this way:

Keflex min/day = 30 min/1 dose x 2 doses/day = 60 min. = 1 hour

Now, the other two antibiotics:

Cipro min/day = 30 min/dose x 3 doses/day = 90 min. = 1.5 hr.

Levaquin min/day = 60 min/dose x 1 dose/day = 60 min. = 1 hr.

Then we add the total time during a 24 hour period that secondary fluids are running in: 1 + 1.5 + 1 = 3.5 hours.

So the LR does not run in for 24 hours a day, because for 3.5 hours a day, secondary fluids are running. Thus, the LR runs 24 - 3.5 = 20.5 hours a day. How much LR runs in 24 hours, then?

LR 125 ml/hr x 20.5 hr = 2562.5 ml

You then add the total volume for the four fluids together for the 24 hour total:

2562.5 ml (LR)

+ 600 ml (secondary fluids)

3162.5 ml total 24 hour IV intake.

All this can be abbreviated, as follows:

| LR | | Keflex | | Cipro | | Levaquin | |
|---|---|---|---|---|---|---|---|
| 125 ml/hr | | 100 ml/dose | | 50 ml/dose | | 250 ml/dose | |
| X 20.5 hr | | x 2 doses | | x 3 doses | | x 1 dose | |
| 2562.5 ml | + | 200 ml | + | 150 ml | + | 250 ml | = **3162.5 ml** |
| 24-3.5 = 20.5 hr | - | 1 hr | - | 1.5 hr | - | 1 hr | |

# IV RECONSTITUTION PROBLEMS

You may want to review how you did reconstitution problems for 101 math. Initially, for IV problems, you do it exactly the same way: usually, concentration of the medication times the doctor's order in determining the desired dose. In IV math, what is affected by reconstituting medications is the flow rate, because the amount in the bag to be infused is changed when medication is added to the bag.

## Example 1

The order is to reconstitute an antibiotic to create a concentration of 1000 mg in 100 ml. It is available in a 5 ml vial containing 250 mg per ml. How much fluid must you add to reach the desired concentration? (Concentration: 250 mg/ml. Doctor's order: 1000 mg. *Note that the bag size of 100 ml does not enter your computations at this point!*)

ml = 1 ml/250 mg x 1000 mg/d.o. = 4 ml

The doctor has ordered 1000 mg of the medication to be given over 30 minutes twice daily. What would the flow rate be?

*How much fluid will you be giving to give the 1000 mg? Remember, the medication was added to the bag, so you now have 100 ml + 4 ml = 104 ml!*

ml/hr = 104 ml/1000 mg x 1000 mg/30 min x 60 min/hr = 208 ml/hr

Note the flow rate is the concentration of the medication x the doctor's order. *This is true only when the doctor has ordered infusion in something other than ml/hr, in this particular example, in mg/hr.*

Suppose the previous example had been worded somewhat differently, by combining the two parts of the problem:

The order is to reconstitute an antibiotic to create a concentration of 100 mg in 100 ml. It is available in a 5 ml vial containing 250 mg/ml. The doctor has ordered 1000 mg of the medication to be given over 30 minutes twice daily. What flow rate would you set on the pump to infuse this medication?

This is the <u>same problem as given in example 1</u>. *Note that this problem <u>cannot</u> be solved in a single step or a single equation. It <u>must</u> be done in two steps,* because you must first determine how much fluid has been added to the 100 ml bag before you can calculate the correct flow rate to set.

Let's look at another, similar example.

## Example 2

The medication comes 400 mg/2 ml. You are to give 1 g. How much would you add to a 100 ml bag of D5NS to achieve the desired concentration of 1 g/100 ml?

ml = 2 ml/400 mg x 1000 mg/1 g x 1 g/d.o. = 5 ml

Flow rate to give it over 45 minutes?

ml/hr = 105 ml/45 min x 60 min/hr = 140 ml/hr

Again, this problem could be combined: The medication comes 400 mg/2 ml. You are to give 1 g in a 100 ml bag of D5NS. What flow rate would you set to infuse the medication in 45 minutes?

Again, as in the previous example, this problem <u>must</u> be done in two steps. First, you must determine how much has been added to the D5NS bag (namely, the 5 ml we just calculated), and only then can you determine the flow rate to set (the 140 ml/hr above).

# IV DOSAGE CALCULATIONS

1.  Your patient is to receive 3 liters of maintenance fluids in the next 12 hours. At what rate should you set the pump?

2.  Using 15 gtt/ml tubing, what would the drip rate be for problem 1?

3.  What tubing (macro or micro) would you use for each of the following?

    a.  A frail 72-year-old female with fluids ordered at 75 ml/hr
    b.  A 27-year-old male with pneumonia who is to get antibiotics at 100 ml/hr
    c.  A 10-year-old child with normal saline ordered at 60 ml/hr
    d.  A 42-year-old post-surgical patient receiving a blood transfusion

4.  Your patient is to receive the full dose of 250 ml of an antibiotic within the two-hour window prior to his scheduled surgery. Surgery is scheduled for noon. You therefore hang the antibiotic at 1000 at 125 ml an hour. At 1045, the patient has to be disconnected from his IV for an MRI. He does not return until 1115. At what rate do you have to set the pump now to ensure all of the antibiotic will be infused prior to the patient's scheduled surgery time?

5.  Mr. Lawler has 900 ml of NS to infuse at 85 ml/hr. How long will it take to infuse?

6.  What hourly dosage of heparin will your patient receive if he is getting the usual 100:1 (25,000 units/250 ml) heparin at 14.7 ml/hr?

7.  Calculate the flow rate and drip rate for a patient receiving 400 ml in two and a half hours. Tubing available is 20 gtt/ml.

8.  The patient has 500 ml to be infused in 6 hours. Calculate the drip rate, using 15 gtt/ml tubing.

9.  Ms. Snowden is to get 4 mg of a medication per Kg of body weight. She weighs 159 pounds. The medication is then to be diluted in 150 ml NS and infused at 26 mg/hr. What is the hourly rate?

10. Mr. Peterson is very ill. He has D5W infusing at 100 ml/hr. The doctor has also ordered levofloxacin 1 g in 250 ml D5W twice daily, to infuse over 90 minutes, Ancef 1.5 g in 150 ml every eight hours, to infuse over an hour, and Aztreonam 1 g in 100 ml every six hours, to infuse over 30 minutes. Calculate the flow rate for each of the antibiotics, and determine Mr. Peterson's 24-hour parenteral intake.

11. What is the needed hourly rate if 100 ml is to be infused in 35 minutes?

12. Your patient is receiving a magnesium rider at 25 ml/hr. The concentration of the rider is 5 g in 100 ml. What is his hourly dosage?

13. Mr. Aaronson is to receive 2 L of D5 1/2 NS over the next 12 hours. What will the hourly rate be?

14. Mr. Franklin is receiving his IV medication at 200 mg/hr. He is receiving 2 g of the medication in 250 ml of NS. Another medication is to be hung as soon as the current medication is completely infused. It is now 1400. At what time should you be able to hang the new medication?

15. Determine the flow rate needed to infuse the medication in the previous problem in half the time you calculated for the problem.

16. The medication is infusing at 75 ml/hr. Calculate the drip rate separately using 10, 15, 20, and 60 gtt/ml tubing.

**Questions 17 – 19 are based on the following scenario:**

**Your patient is to receive one liter of IV fluids over 12 hours. You hang the bag at 0200. When you check the bag at 0530, you realize only 380 ml have infused.**

17. What flow rate should have been set per the original order?

18. At what flow rate was it actually infusing?

19.   At what rate should you now set the pump to be sure the one liter finishes infusing at 1400?

20.   Mr. Anodin is to receive 700 ml of fluid at 45 ml/hr. How long will it require to infuse?

21.   Calculate the flow rate and drip rate for a 100 ml dose of a medication which is to infuse in 25 minutes.

22.   Mr. Baker has orders for maintenance fluids to infuse one liter every 9 hours. You hang a fresh one-liter bag at 0700. At 0900, Mr. Baker leaves the floor for a test. You assume his IV has gone with him and do not realize until two hours and 15 minutes after he returns at 0945 that he was disconnected from his IV fluids and never reconnected. At what rate must you now set the pump to meet the 9-hour infusion deadline for this bag of fluid?

23. The doctor has ordered a medication which comes in a vial with a concentration of 350 mg/ml. You are to add 2.1 g of this medication to a 100 ml bag of NS and infuse it in 30 min. At what rate will you set the pump?

24. 750 ml of fluid is infusing at 33 gtt/min using 15 gtt/ml tubing. What is its flow rate?

25. Heparin 10,000 units in 100 ml is infusing at 12.9 ml/hr. What is the hourly dosage?

26. You are to reconstitute 1 g of a powdered medication with 20 ml of sterile water. How much of this reconstituted medication will you add to a 100 ml bag of D5W to create the doctor's order of 250 mg of the medication?

27. In the previous problem, what flow rate would you set to give 40 mg/hour?

28. Mrs. Jackson is receiving D5 1/2 NS at 150 ml/hr, antibiotic A 500 mg in 50 ml every six hours (infuse over 30 minutes), antibiotic B 2 g in 150 ml three times daily (infuse over one hour), and a potassium rider of 200 ml (infuse over 90 minutes). She is on strict I&O. What is her 24-hour parenteral intake?

29. With 10 gtt/ml tubing, determine flow rate and drip rate for each of the fluids in the previous problem.

30. The patient is to receive a 75 ml dose of medication IV at 128.6 ml/hr. How many minutes will it take to infuse?

31. It is now 0835. Your patient has 700 ml of fluid left in a bag running at 55 ml/hr. At what time will the bag be empty?

32. After reconstituting a medication, you have a 10 ml vial containing 500 mg of medication per 2 ml. The doctor has ordered 750 mg of medication be given. How much of the reconstituted medication will you need to use?

33. In the previous problem, you add the needed amount of reconstituted medication to a 50 ml bag. What flow rate will you set to infuse it in 30 minutes?

34. The patient is to receive 100 ml of fluid in 40 minutes. Calculate the flow rate and drip rate.

35. The patient has 500 ml of fluid to be infused, using 15 gtt/ml tubing and running at 40 gtt/min. How long will it take to infuse?

36. Heparin is infusing at 9.8 ml/hr. The solution infusing has 10,000 units heparin in 100 ml D5W. What is the hourly dosage?

**Questions 37 and 38 are based on the following:**

**The antibiotic is to be reconstituted to create a concentration of 500 mg in 100 ml. The available antibiotic comes in a 5 ml vial containing 2 g.**

37. How much of the available antibiotic must be added to the 100 ml bag to create the desired concentration? (Take your answer to hundredths.)

38. At what rate would you set the pump for the newly reconstituted medication to infuse in 45 minutes?

39. It is 0800. There are 720 ml remaining in the bag of ½ NS, which is infusing at 70 ml/hr. At what time will you need to hang a new bag, assuming you let the old bag run until empty?

40. If a patient has 50 ml to infuse in 25 minutes, at what rate should you set the pump?

41. A liter of D5.2NS is to infuse at 42 gtt/min, using tubing labeled 20 gtt/ml. How long will it take to infuse?

42. 250 ml of a medication are to be infused in one hour. The set is calibrated at 15 gtt/ml. What is the drip rate?

**Questions 43 and 44 are based on the following information:**

**Available medication is 1.5 g in a 10 ml vial. The doctor has ordered a 600 mg dose.**

43. How much should you add to the 100 ml bag of D5W to create the ordered dose?

44. What flow rate would you set if the medication is to infuse in 30 minutes?

45. A liter of D5.45NS is to infuse in eleven hours. Calculate the flow rate and drip rate. Only microdrip tubing is available.

46. The doctor has ordered a 500 ml bolus of NS. It will infuse at 60 gtt/min, using 20 gtt/ml tubing. How long will it take to infuse?

47. In the previous problem, what is the flow rate?

48. The patient is on strict I&O. In the past 24 hours, he has had emesis of 380 ml and diarrhea of 650 ml. You are now to calculate his parenteral intake over the same period of time. He is receiving D5W at 125 ml/hr, antibiotic A 2 g in 150 ml every eight hours (infused over 60 minutes) and antibiotic B 500 mg in 50 ml every six hours (infused over 30 minutes). What is his 24- hour parenteral intake?

49. A patient is to receive a 500 ml bolus of fluid over a 3-hour period just prior to surgery scheduled at 1100. You hang the bag at 0745. At 0930 the IV is discontinued as the patient is taken from the floor for an Xray, returning at 1015. At what rate should you restart the IV fluids to ensure complete infusion by 1100?

50. 1000 ml of LR is infusing at 60 gtt/min using tubing labeled 20 gtt/ml. How long will it take for complete infusion?

51. Calculate the flow rate and drip rate necessary to infuse 500 ml of IV fluids in two and one half hours. Tubing is calibrated at 10 gtt/ml.

52. The antibiotic comes as 2 g powder in a 10 ml vial. You are to reconstitute it using 8 ml of sterile water, then add it to a 50 ml bag of D5W to meet the doctor's order. The order is for 500 mg of the antibiotic every 8 hours. How much of the reconstituted fluid will you add to the bag?

53. Your patient is receiving D5 1/2 NS at 180 ml/hr. The doctor has also ordered two antibiotics: antibiotic A 500 mg in 50 ml every 6 hours (infuse over 30 min.), and antibiotic B 1.5 g in 100 ml every 8 hours (infuse over 60 min.). How much IV fluid will infuse in 24 hours?

54. For the three IV fluids in the previous problem, what are the flow rate and drip rate of each? Tubing size: 15 gtt/ml.

55. Your patient is to receive 2 liters of fluid overnight, all to be infused prior to surgery scheduled for 0900 tomorrow morning. You hang the first liter bag at 2000 and the infusion is complete at 0200. You hang the second liter bag immediately (at 0200). At 0515 the pump alarms, and you note the site has infiltrated at some point with only 450 ml infused. By the time you start a new IV site and restart the infusion, it is 0545.

    a.   At what rate did the first liter bag infuse?

    b.   At what rate will you need to set the pump at 0545 to be sure the second liter is infused prior to surgery?

56. You hang a 500 ml bolus at 0700, to infuse at 135 ml/hr. At what time will the bag be empty?

57. The liter bag of Lactated Ringer's is infusing at 22 gtt/min using 20 gtt/ml tubing. How long will it take to infuse?

58. The medication comes in a 10 ml vial with a concentration of 120 mg/ml. The doctor's order is for 1 g in 100 ml to be given over 90 min.

    a.    How much of the medication will need to be added to the 100 ml bag to follow the order?

    b.    At what rate will you infuse the medication?

59. Calculate the flow rate for the following:

    a.    50 ml in 15 minutes

    b.    100 ml in 45 minutes

    c.    250 ml in 90 minutes

60. The pharmacy sent up three antibiotics, all scheduled to be hung at 0900. The protocol at your facility states all fluids must be administered within 45 minutes of their scheduled time. The fluids ordered are A, to infuse over 90 minutes; B, to infuse over 60 minutes; and C, to infuse over 30 minutes. At what time would you hang each to follow facility policy?

61. The ordered medication is available in a 10 ml vial containing 500 mg/ml. The doctor has ordered 3.5 g in 250 ml ½ NS to be infused over 90 minutes, using 10 gtt/ml tubing.

    a.    How much medication will you add to the NS?

    b.    At what rate will you set the pump?

    c.    What would the drip rate be?

62. The liter bag of D5 1/2 NS is infusing at 85 ml/hr. The nurse on the previous shift states she just hung it at 0530. At what time should you be prepared to hang a new bag?

63. The patient is receiving NS at 150 ml an hour. He has a 50 ml potassium rider ordered (to infuse over 90 minutes), a 50 ml magnesium rider (to infuse over 30 minutes) and two antibiotics. Antibiotic A 500 mg in 100 ml is ordered every 8 hours (to infuse over 30 minutes), and antibiotic B 1 g in 200 ml is ordered every 12 hours (to infuse over 90 minutes). Total 24- hour parenteral intake?

64. Calculate the drip rate for the following:

   a.   1000 ml infusing in 12 hours

   b.   750 ml infusing in 6 hours

   c.   150 ml infusing in 90 minutes

65. The doctor has ordered 1500 ml of fluid infused within 10 hours. You hang the fluid at 1000. At 1230 the patient's IV is disconnected and he leaves the floor for testing, not returning until 1430. You reconnect his IV immediately. At what rate should you set the pump now, to comply with the order?

66. The patient has a heparin drip 25,000 units in 250 ml, infusing at 1320 units per hour. What is the flow rate?

67. A liter bag of D5W is infusing at 34 gtt/min using 15 gtt/ml tubing. What is the flow rate?

68. In the previous problem, how long will it take to infuse?

69. Calculate flow rate and drip rate for 250 ml to infuse in 45 minutes.

70. Your patient has a loading dose of a medication 1500 mg in 250 ml, to infuse in 90 minutes. What is the hourly dosage of this medication?

71. The medication is available 3 g in a 10 ml vial. The doctor has ordered 750 mg be added to a 50 ml bag of D5W and infused every 6 hours (infuse over 30 minutes). How much of the medication should you add to the D5W?

72. Calculate the flow rate and drip rate for the previous problem.

73. At 1100, you hang a liter bolus of NS at 110 ml/hr. At what time will the bolus be complete?

74. The doctor has ordered NS at a KVO (keep vein open) rate of 20 ml/hr. No IV bag may hang for more than 24 hours, per hospital policy. Available bags: 50 ml, 100 ml, 250 ml, 500 ml, and 1 liter. Which would you choose to hang at 0800, so another does not have to be hung for 24 hours? (Assume no other IV fluids, and unbroken flow.)

75. The medication is available in a vial 2 g in 2 ml of fluid. You dilute this with 20 ml of sterile water, then add 1.2 g of it to a 100 ml bag of NS. How much fluid will you add to the bag?

76. Order: 500 ml to infuse in 6 hours. Only tubing available is 20 gtt/ml. What are the flow rate and drip rate?

77. A liter bag of NS is infusing at 41 gtt/min, using 20 gtt/ml tubing. How long will it take to infuse?

78. In the previous problem, at what rate is the pump set?

79. The heparin is available 25,000 units in 250 ml. The doctor has ordered the heparin to be infused at 14.3 ml/hr. What is the patient's hourly dosage?

80. The patient is to get a 750 ml bolus of D5 1/2 NS at 60 ml/hr. If you hang it at 0930, at what time will the ordered amount have infused?

81. Using 20 gtt/ml tubing and running at 42 gtt/min, how long will it take for a one liter bag of IV fluids to infuse?

82. Calculate the flow rate and drip rate of 750 ml infusing in 8 hours. Tubing available: 10 gtt/ml.

83. The IV antibiotic ordered contains 1000 mg in 150 ml, infusing in 45 minutes. What is the hourly dosage?

84. Patient's meds: D5W at 100 ml/hr, antibiotic A 1000 mg in 100 ml twice daily (infuse over 30 minutes), antibiotic B 2.5 g in 150 ml every 8 hours (infuse over 90 minutes). What is his 24-hour parenteral intake?

85. Order: 1 liter LR to be hung at 0900 and infused by the scheduled time of surgery at 1500. At 1200 the patient goes down for an MRI and his IV is disconnected for one hour.

    a.     What was the initial flow rate when you hung the LR?

    b.     What will the adjusted flow rate be at 1300, in order for the infusion to be complete by 1500?

86. Your patient has IV fluids infusing at a KVO rate of 25 ml/hr. Using 15 gtt/ml tubing, calculate the drip rate.

87. 250 ml of an antibiotic has been ordered, to infuse in 90 minutes. Flow rate and drip rate?

88. IV fluids are infusing at 135 ml/hr. Assuming you hung the liter bag of fluids at 0900, at what time will the bag be empty?

89. The patient has D5 1/2 NS infusing at 125 ml/hr. A 50 ml potassium rider is to be given over 1 hour. The patient also has 100 ml of antibiotic A every 6 hours (infuse over 30 minutes) and 200 ml of antibiotic B twice daily (infuse over 60 minutes). What is his 24-hour parenteral intake?

90. What is the drip rate of each IV fluid in the previous problem, using 20 gtt/ml tubing?

91. The doctor has ordered 750 mg of a medication be added to a 50 ml bag of NS and infused over 30 minutes. The medication must be reconstituted. It is available 3 g in a 10 ml vial.

    a. How much of the medication will you add to the 50 ml bag to follow the doctor's order?

    b. At what rate will you set the pump to infuse the medication?

92. Heparin is available 10,000 units in 100 ml of D5W. It is infusing into your patient at 13.6 ml/hr. What is the hourly dosage?

93. A liter of IV fluids is flowing at 26 gtt/min using 15 gtt/ml tubing.

    a.  If you hang the bag at 1130, at what time will you need to hang a new bag? (Assume the old bag is completely empty before a new one is hung.)

    b.  At what flow rate is it infusing?

94. You are to add NS to a vial to create a concentration of 500 mg/ml. The 10 ml vial contains 4 g of a powdered medication. How much fluid do you need to add?

95. A liter bag of fluid is infusing at 90 ml/hr. The only tubing available is 10 gtt/ml. What is the drip rate for this fluid?

96.  750 mg of a medication in 100 ml NS is to infuse at 60 mg/hr. What is the flow rate?

97.  500 ml of D5W is to infuse in 6 hours. What is the drip rate?

98.  You are to infuse 500 ml of D5NS at 130 ml/hr. What is the drip rate

    a.  with 10 gtt/ml tubing?

    b.  with 15 gtt/ml tubing?

    c.  with 20 gtt/ml tubing?

99.  Your medication is available 5 g (5000 mg) in 100 ml. You are to infuse it at 125 ml/hr. What is the hourly dosage?

100. The medication comes in a powdered form with 2 g in a vial. You add 8 ml of sterile water to reconstitute the medication. The MD has ordered 1200 mg of the medication be added to a 100 ml bag which is to be infused over 45 minutes.

    a.    How much of the reconstituted medication will be added to the 100 ml bag?

    b.    What flow rate should you set to infuse the medication in 45 minutes?

101. Order reads 1000 ml D5 1/2 NS in 7 hours. Calculate flow rate and drip rate. The IV set is labeled 15 gtt/ml.

102. Order: 1500 ml NS to infuse at 90 ml/hr. The only tubing available is 20 gtt/ml.

    a.    How long will it take to run in?

    b.    What is the drip rate?

103. The order is for 1500 ml D5W. The drop factor is 15 gtt/ml, and the drip rate is 40 gtt/min. How many hours and minutes will it take to infuse?

104. Heparin is to infuse at 9 ml/hr. The IV solution is 25,000 units heparin in 250 ml D5W. What is the hourly dosage? What is the drip rate?

105. The patient is to receive a heparin drip, concentration 10,000 units/100 ml D5W. It is to infuse at 7.6 ml/hr. What is the hourly dosage, and what is the gtt rate? The only tubing available is 10 gtt/ml.

106. The order is to reconstitute Ancef to create a concentration of 1000 mg in 50 ml. It comes in a vial with 1 g in 2 ml. How much fluid must you add to reach the desired concentration? Then Ancef 1000 mg in 50 ml is to infuse over 45 minutes. What is the flow rate?

107. The patient has acute gastroenteritis, and is on strict I&O. He is receiving LR 125 ml/hr, is getting Flagyl 1 g in 100 ml NS twice a day (infused over 60 minutes), and Ancef 1000 mg in 50 ml D5W every 8 hours (infused over 30 minutes). What is his 24-hour IV input?

108. D5W 2000 ml is to run for 16 hours. The only tubing available is 15 gtt/ml. What is the flow rate? The drip rate?

109. 500 ml 0.2NS is to infuse over 6 hours.

    a.     What tubing should you use?

    b.     What is the drip rate?

110. D5W 1800 ml is ordered, to infuse over 15 hours, using a 15 gtt/ml set. What are the flow rate and drip rate?

111. The order reads: Infuse 50 ml D5W in 40 minutes.

    a.     Tubing size?

    b.     Flow rate?

    c.    Drip rate?

112.  1 L D5W is to infuse at 33 gtt/min using a 15 gtt/ml set. How long will it take to infuse?

113.  Order: Transfuse 500 ml whole blood at 150 ml/hr. The transfusion was started at 1440.

    a.    How long will it take to infuse?

    b.    What will be the completion time?

114.  The MD orders 3500 ml D5.2NS to be given over the next 18 hours. Calculate the hourly and drip rate.

115.  Levaquin 250 mg IV in 50 ml D5W is to be infused in one hour. What is the drip rate?

116. An IV of 500 ml D5W is to infuse in 6 hours. The only tubing available is 10 gtt/ml. What is the drip rate?

117. D5W 2000 ml is to run in 16 hours. The set calibration is 10 gtt/ml. What is the drip rate?

118. LR at 80 ml/hr is hung. What is the drip rate, and how much fluid will the patient get over the next 24 hours?

119. Aminophylline 28 mg/hr is to be given to the patient IV. Available is aminophylline 500 mg in ½ L D5W. What is the hourly rate to be given, and what is the drip rate?

120. Cipro is available 1 g in a 2.6 ml vial. The doctor wants the patient to receive a 400 mg dose. How much fluid should you add to the 100 ml bag of D5W? Cipro 400 mg in 100 ml D5W is to infuse over 1 hour. Drip rate?

121. You are to give 1500 ml NS in 12 hours. Calculate the hourly and drip rate.

122. 1 liter of D5W is to infuse at 125 ml per hour. How long will it take to run in?

123. Aminophylline is ordered at 23 mg per hour. It is available 1 g in 500 ml of NS. What is the flow rate at which you will set the pump? What is the drip rate?

124. Heparin has been mixed at 10,000 units in a 100 ml bag of NS. It is to infuse at 12 ml per hour. What is the hourly dosage?

125. 1 liter of D5 1/2 NS is to infuse over 12 hours. What is the flow rate? The drip rate? Tubing available: 15 gtt/ml.

126. You have been asked to keep input/output on a patient. He is NPO (getting nothing by mouth), but is on D5W at 125 ml/hr, and is also getting three antibiotics: Levaquin 250 mg in 100 ml (infused over 1 hour) daily, Keflex 500 mg in 250 ml (infused over 1 hour) three times a day, and Cipro 1 g in 150 ml (infused over 1 hour) twice a day. What is the total IV input in 24 hours?

127. The dehydrated patient is to get 500 ml over the next 90 minutes. At what rate will you set the pump?

128. The doctor has ordered 2 liters of LR to be given to the patient during the next 15 hours. What is the drip rate?

129. There are 380 ml left in the IV bag. It is now 1400. The patient has a test scheduled at 1700. At what rate should you set the pump to be sure the infusion is complete before the test?

130. 250 ml of NS was started at 0900, infusing at 48 gtt/min and using 15 gtt/ml tubing. How long will it take to infuse? What will the flow rate be?

131. Calculate the drip rate for 50 ml of Ancef to infuse over 30 minutes. Then calculate the drip rate for 100 ml of Zithromycin to infuse over 60 minutes.

132. 750 ml of D5LR is running at 40 gtt/min with a 15 gtt/ml tubing set. What is its infusion rate? How long will it take to finish running?

133. 500 mg of Zosyn in 100 ml NS is to infuse at 60 mg per hour. What is the flow rate? The drip rate?

134. Using IV tubing with a drop factor of 15 gtt/ml, and an order for 250 ml NS to be given over 8 hours, calculate the flow rate and drip rate.

135. 50 ml of an antibiotic is to be infused in 20 minutes. What is the flow rate? What tubing size will you use?

136. The patient has an oncology drug prescribed. The doctor orders 15 mg/kg/day, in four divided doses. The patient weighs 157 pounds. How much will the patient receive per dose?

137. If a medication comes 500 mg/250 ml, and each dose is to infuse in 45 minutes, what flow rate will you set for each dose?

138. The doctor has ordered the dehydrated patient to receive 3 liters of LR in the next 16 hours. Calculate the flow rate and drip rate.

139. Your patient has a 500 ml bolus of NS to be infused at 125 ml/hr. How long will it take to infuse?

140. Calculate the drip rate of 1 liter of D5 1/2 NS infusing at 140 ml/hr, using:

    a.    10 gtt/ml tubing

    b.    15 gtt/ml tubing

    c.    20 gtt/ml tubing

141. The flow rate of your patient's medication is 160 ml/hr. What is the drip rate?

142. Available: 3 g in 2 ml NS, to be added to a 100 ml bag of NS
Order: Give at 700 mg/hr
Flow rate?

143. The medication comes in a 10 ml vial containing 0.5 g/ml. The doctor has ordered 2 g in 100 ml D5W.

    a.    How much medication will you add to the bag?

b.    What flow rate will you set to infuse it in 30 minutes?

144. The ordered medication is available 250 mg/ml. You are to give 2 g in a 100 ml bag of D5NS. What rate would you set on the pump to infuse it in 45 minutes?

145. You hang 250 ml of medicine at 0900, using 15 gtt/ml tubing and a drip rate of 26 gtt/min. At what time will the bag be empty?

146. Heparin 25,000 units in 250 ml NS is infusing at 13.7 ml/hr. Calculate the drip rate.

147. 500 ml of NS is infusing at 35 gtt/min using 20 gtt/ml tubing. Calculate the flow rate.

148. You add 8 ml of sterile water to reconstitute 2 g of a powdered medication. The doctor's order is to give 1.5 g of the medication in 100 ml of NS over 1 hour.

    a.    How much fluid will you add to the 100 ml bag?

    b.    What flow rate will you set to infuse the medication?

149. 30 mEq of potassium in 100 ml 0.45NS is infusing over 90 minutes. What is the hourly dosage?

150. Your patient is to receive a medication at 12 mg/Kg, which is to be added to a 100 ml bag of NS and to infuse at 38 mg/hr. The patient weighs 118.8 lb. Calculate the flow rate.

# PEDIATRIC DOSAGE CALCULATIONS

# PEDIATRIC MATH

A child is not the same patient as an adult. Not only do we have no idea what a child's response may be to a medication new to them, but the dose must be adjusted to allow for the enormous variety in size of pediatric patients, from the tiny 2.5 pound premature infant to the 17-year-old high school student. There are two ways in which pediatric doses allow for this: dose is based on the child's weight (mg per Kg), or on the child's $M^2$.

It is your responsibility as the nurse to be sure the dose you are going to give is safe for the child.

So let's look first at how to calculate the size of the child's body, using the $M^2$.

## $M^2$ formula

$$\frac{\sqrt{\text{Wt in Kg x ht in cm}}}{3600}$$

**NOTE:** *If pt information is given in inches and pounds, it must be converted to metric for these calculations.*

The $M^2$ formula gives the body surface area. $M^2$ is meters squared.

Now, a basic rule.

## Basic rules

**If your problem gives you a range** for the medication dosage, utilize that range in determining whether or not a doctor's order is safe for the pediatric patient.

**If the problem gives you no range**, the doctor's order must be the dose you have calculated, or it is considered unsafe. Any time the order is unsafe, you would have to call the MD and get a revision of the order.

[There are areas of pediatric medical care (such as pediatric oncology) in which some faculties may allow you to give the dose if it falls between 90 and 110% of the original order – that is, the doctor's order plus or minus 10 percent, and any number within that range would be considered a safe dose. However, do not assume this is the case at your facility, without further instructions!]

## Rounding

Because small changes in dose can have a large impact on a tiny pediatric patient, we want all calculations to be as precise as possible. Therefore, in doing pediatric dosage calculations, we will take all answers to three places (thousandths) and round them to two places (hundredths).

## Some further information:

If a patient's size is given in feet and inches, you must still use inches only to calculate the M². Say your patient's height is given as 3'4" (three feet four inches). Using your conversion factor, you can calculate

$$\text{inches} = \frac{12 \text{ inches}}{1 \text{ foot}} \times 3 \text{ feet} = 36 \text{ inches}$$

But the patient is 3 feet four inches tall, or 36 + 4 = 40 inches tall. You can now correctly calculate your M², converting the inches into cm.

If a patient's weight is given in lb and oz (pounds and ounces), you must convert it to lb to calculate the M². Say your patient's weight is 6 lb 9 oz. Again, use your conversion factor to determine what portion of a lb the 9 oz is. Your patient weighs 6 lb plus 9/16 lb (since a lb = 16 oz). Now turn this into a decimal:

$$\text{lb} = \frac{1 \text{ lb}}{16 \text{ oz}} \times 9 \text{ oz} = 0.56 \text{ lb, so your patient weighs 6.56 lb.}$$

You can now convert this to Kg and proceed with your calculations.

Now let's look at a couple of other areas for which you will have pediatric problems: maintenance fluids, and NG replacement fluids.

# MAINTENANCE FLUID PROBLEMS

The doctor may order the child to receive maintenance fluids. The order is based on the child's weight: the more the child weighs, the more fluid they receive over a 24-hour period. The usual order is as follows (the 100-50-20 order):

**100 ml/kg for the first 10 kg of the child's weight**

**50 ml/kg for the next 10 kg of the child's weight**

**20 ml/kg for every kg or portion of a kg of the child's weight over 20 kg**

## How to solve maintenance fluid problems

1. Look at this order for a moment. If a child weighs less than 10 kg, only the first portion of the order pertains. For a child weighing 8.8 kg, then:

$$\frac{100 \text{ ml}}{\text{kg}} \times 8.8 \text{ kg} = 880 \text{ ml, to be given over 24 hours}$$

2. Bring the second part of the order in for a larger child. Say the child weighs 14 kg. The first portion of the maintenance will always be the same:

$$\frac{100 \text{ ml}}{\text{kg}} \times 10 \text{ kg} = 1000 \text{ ml}$$

Now add the second part of the order for the balance of the child's weight: 14 kg less the 10 kg already dealt with by the first portion of the order leaves 4 kg.

$$\frac{50 \text{ ml}}{\text{kg}} \times 4 \text{ kg} = 200 \text{ ml}$$

so the patient will receive 1000 ml + 200 ml = 1200 ml over 24 hours.

3. For a child weighing more than 20 kg, you will need to utilize all three parts of the

maintenance order, as shown below for a child weighing 39 kg:

$$\frac{100 \text{ ml}}{\text{kg}} \times 10 \text{ kg} = 1000 \text{ ml}$$

$$\frac{50 \text{ ml}}{\text{kg}} \times 10 \text{ kg} = 500 \text{ ml}$$

So we have accounted for the first 20 kg of the child's weight. Notice that for the first 20 kg of any patient's weight, the total will always be the same: 1000 ml + 500 ml = 1500 ml

Now we must deal with the remainder of the patient's weight. The child weighed 39 kg. We have dealt with the first 20 kg, so 39 − 20 = 19 kg remaining.

$$\frac{20 \text{ ml}}{\text{kg}} \times 19 \text{ kg} = 380 \text{ ml}$$

So this child's total maintenance fluid will be 1000 + 500 + 380 ml = 1880 ml over 24 hours.

## Example 1

The doctor has ordered maintenance fluids for your 24.5 kg patient, using the usual 100-50-20 order. How much fluid should the patient receive in the next 24 hours?

100 ml/kg x 10 kg  =  1000 ml

50 ml/kg x 10 kg  =  500 ml

20 ml/kg x 4.5 kg  =  <u>90 ml</u>

                             1590 ml

**NOTE:** The doctor may also order some variant of the basic maintenance fluid order. For example, he may order ½ maintenance fluids, or 1.5 x maintenance fluids. You then calculate the basic maintenance fluid amount, and multiply it, for example, by 0.5 or 1.5, depending on the doctor's order.

# Example 2

The doctor has ordered 1.5x maintenance fluids for your 48.6 kg patient. How much should your patient receive in the next 24 hours?

100 ml/kg x 10 kg = 1000 ml

50 ml/kg x 10 kg = 500 ml

20 ml/kg x 28.6 kg = 572 ml for a total of 2072 ml. But the order is for 1.5x maintenance, so your answer must be 2072 x 1.5 = 3108 ml

# BOLUS FLUIDS

## Bolus fluids

A patient may be admitted who is suffering from dehydration. This may be the result of a variety of causes: exposure to heat, lack of intake of fluid, vomiting, diarrhea. The cause doesn't matter. What does matter is that the doctor will probably not only order IV fluids, he may well also order a bolus given. The order might be written; 1L normal saline given over four hours, then D5NS at 100 ml/hr.

This would be treated like any other IV problem: how much is ordered, and over what period of time, to determine the flow rate you must set for the bolus. In the example above:

1000ml/4 hr = 250 ml per hour. Then the IV fluid would need to be changed, and the flow rate reduced according to the doctor's orders.

# NG REPLACEMENT FLUIDS

An adult may not be bothered much by NG tube suctioning, unless the volume suctioned is very great. However, even small amounts lost to the NG by small children can be significant, and may need to be replaced.

The doctor will write orders for the replacement, and may well order a fluid with electrolytes to help replace those lost to the NG. If so, the replacement fluid may or may not be the same as the IV fluid the patient has running. If it is the same fluid, simply take the amount suctioned the previous shift, divide it by 12, and add that to the flow rate for the fluid infusing, as in the following problem.

## Example 1

The patient has D5 1/2 NS with 20 mEq of potassium running at 50 ml an hour. He had 120 ml of fluid suctioned out in the previous 12-hour shift. At what rate should you set the pump in order to continue the ordered infusion plus replace the fluid suctioned with D5 1/2 NS with 20 mEq KCl?

120 ml/12 hr = 10 ml/hr for replacement of fluid lost to the NG

Current infusion rate = 50 ml/hr + 10 ml/hr = 60 ml/hr

What if the replacement fluid ordered is not the same as that currently infusing? Then you would simply run the replacement fluid in separately. *This cannot be done as a piggyback, because the primary fluid would stop while the piggyback ran in.* It could be done through a Y-site, so both fluids could run in at the same time, through a separate IV site, through a separate pump, or through another port of the same central line.

## Example 2

Your pediatric patient has had gastric surgery and now has an NG tube to low wall suction. This tube has suctioned 50 ml on the last shift. Your orders are to replace the drainage with D5 1/2 NS with 20 mEq KCl over 12 hours. The current peripheral IV is D5W infusing at 40 ml/hr.

50ml/12 hr = 4.2 ml per hour for the replacement fluid, while the primary fluid ordered would continue to infuse at 40 ml/hr. Your choices for how to do this are given above.

Another possibility for your pediatric patient: The doctor might order peripheral IV to run in at the fluid maintenance rate (or some multiple thereof), rather than giving a set rate in his order.

## Example 3

The doctor ordered NG replacement fluid (D5 1/2 NS with 20 mEq of KCl over 12 hours) for 100 ml suctioned out the previous shift. The child weighs 50 pounds and is 38 inches tall. His regular IV fluid is D5W with multivitamins, to run at 1.5x the fluid maintenance rate. What rate would you set for each fluid?

| Replacement fluid: | 100ml/12 hr | = | 8.3 ml/hr | |
| Regular fluid: | 100ml/kg x 10 kg | = | 1000 ml | (50 lb = 22.73 kg) |
| | 50 ml/kg x 10 kg | = | 500 ml | |
| | 20 ml/kg x 2.73 kg | = | 54.6 ml | |
| | | | 1554.6 ml | |
| | | X | 1.5 | |
| | 2331.9 ml over 24 hours | = | 97.2 ml/hr | |

# PEDIATRIC DOSAGE CALCULATIONS

1.  Your patient weighs 11.4 Kg. According to the literature, the safe dose is 25 to 40 mg/Kg/day in four divided doses. The doctor has ordered 100 mg per dose. Is his order safe?

2.  Your source indicates the safe range is 20 – 30 mg/Kg/day in two divided doses. The medication is available 50 mg/ml. The doctor has ordered 75 mg per dose. The patient weighs 18 lb.

    a.  Is the doctor's order safe?

    b.  How much would you give, in ml, according to the doctor's order?

3.  The doctor has ordered maintenance fluids on your 27.82 Kg pediatric patient. At what rate will you set the pump to give these fluids over the next 24 hours?

4.  The child is to receive 20 mg of a medication per dose, by MD order. Your source states the medication is safe at 50 mg/day in three divided doses. What is the safe dose? And is the doctor's order safe?

5.  What is the $M^2$ for a child who weighs 22.4 Kg and is 50.8 cm tall?

6.  The doctor has ordered 1.5 x maintenance fluids for a child weighing 41.6 Kg.

    a.  How much fluid will the child get in 24 hours?

    b.  Given over a 24-hour period, at what rate would you set the pump to infuse this fluid?

7.  Your 4-year-old, 35 lb. dehydrated patient has a bolus dose of 500 ml of NS to be infused over 4 hours, after which he is to receive 0.45NS at 3.8 ml/Kg/hr.

    a.  What hourly rate will you set for the bolus dose?

    b.  At what rate will the 0.45NS infuse?

8.  Your patient has D5NS infusing at 45 ml/hr. She also has an NG tube, which has drained 110 ml in the previous 12-hour shift. The doctor has ordered D5NS NG replacement fluids. At what rate should you set the pump to comply with the doctor's orders?

9.  What is the M² for a child who is 33 inches tall and weighs 42 lb?

10. The literature indicates a safe dose of a medication is 12 to 35 mg/M². For the patient in problem 9, the doctor has ordered 60 mg/day in six divided doses. Is his order safe?

11. Your source states the medication's safe dose is 3.5 mg/Kg. Your patient weighs 69 lb. The doctor has ordered 120 mg. Is the order safe?

12. Your patient's NG tube drained 138 ml during the previous shift. The patient has ½ NS infusing at 30 ml/hr. The doctor has ordered replacement fluids of D5 1/2 NS. At what rate will you set the pump to replace the fluid lost to the NG tube?

13. A medication has been ordered for an infant at 3 mg/Kg. The child weighs 5 lb 7 oz. How much will you give?

14. A medication is cited in the literature as being safe at 8 – 20 mg/M². Your patient's M² is 0.98. What is the maximum dose you could safely give?

15. The doctor has ordered maintenance fluids under the 100-50-20 protocol for a child weighing 49 Kg. How much fluid will the child receive over the next 24 hours, per the doctor's order?

16. The dehydrated teenager is to receive a one-liter bolus of D5NS over 6 hours, and then to continue D5NS at 125 ml/hr. How much IV fluid will he receive in the next 24 hours?

17. The child weighs 13.6 Kg. The medication is to be given at 20 – 30 mg/Kg/day in four divided doses. What is the safe range per dose?

18. The medication is available in vials with a concentration of 300 mg/5 ml. You are to dilute 175 mg of the medication in a 100 ml bag of D5W. How much of the medication will you add to the bag?

19. For the previous problem, at what rate would you set the pump if the child weighs 1.59 Kg and is to receive 2 mg/Kg/min. of the medication?

20. Calculate the $M^2$ for a patient who weighs 28.7 Kg and is 34.3 cm tall.

21. If the recommended child's dose is 4 – 12 mg/$M^2$, what is the safe dose range for the patient whose $M^2$ you just calculated in problem 20?

22. The doctor has ordered 1.5 x maintenance fluids for a child weighing 39.8 Kg. At what rate would you set a pump to infuse these fluids over 24 hours?

23. Your 8-year-old post-surgical patient has an NG tube which drained 231 ml during the previous shift. The patient has D5 1/2 NS infusing at 35 ml/hr. The doctor has ordered D5 1/2 NS as replacement fluid. At what rate will you set the pump to infuse the lost fluid over the next 12 hours?

24. The order is for 300 mg every 6 hours. The patient weighs 43.7 Kg. The safe range in the literature is 20 – 50 mg/Kg/day in three divided doses. Is the order safe?

25. The doctor has ordered 50 mg of a medication for the child. Your patient weighs 12.3 Kg. The literature states the medication is safe at 6 mg/Kg.

    a. What is the safe dose for this child?

    b. Is the doctor's order safe?

26. The order is for 5.8 mg/Kg/day in three divided doses. Your patient weighs 18.2 Kg, and the medication comes 150 mg/50 ml. How many ml will the child receive per dose?

27. Post-surgery, your three-year-old patient has an NG tube with drainage of 173 ml during the last shift. He has D5LR running at 60 ml/hr. The doctor orders replacement fluids of D5.45NS with 10 mEq of KCl which (after some quick calculations with the NG output) he orders to run at 74.4 ml/hr. Is he correct? If not, why not?

28. Your 34 lb patient is to receive 150 mg of a medication every six hours. The safe range is 25 – 50 mg/Kg/day in divided doses. Is the order a safe dose for the child?

29. The doctor has ordered twice maintenance fluids for your 27 Kg patient. After calculating, he orders them to run at 68.33 ml/hr for the next 24 hours. Are his calculations correct?

30. Referenced pediatric dosage is 25 mg/kg/day. What is a safe daily dose for your newborn 6.36 Kg patient?

31. What is the M$^2$ for a patient who is 4 ft. 10 in. and 102 lb?

32. The literature states the safe range for the medication is 18 – 25 mg/M$^2$ per day in two divided doses. Using the M$^2$ from problem 31, what is the safe range per dose?

33. For the patient in problem 31, another medication is to be given at 30 mg per M$^2$ per day. What daily dose should the patient receive of this medication?

34. The child has IV fluids infusing at 40 ml/hr. The doctor has ordered a 500 ml bolus to be given over six hours, to be added to the current IV fluids. At what rate will you set the pump during that six-hour period?

35. The baby weighs 8 lb 13 oz. The safe dose of the medication order is 40 mg/Kg/day in three divided doses. What is the safe dose per day for this child? Safe dose per dose?

36. Your 18-month-old patient has lost 106 ml in NG drainage in the past 12 hours. What flow rate will you set for the child's replacement fluids?

37.  The order is for 300 mg of an antibiotic to be given in 100 ml of D5.45NS over 40 minutes three times daily. Your reference indicates a safe dose is 20 – 40 mg/Kg/day in two divided doses. Your patient weighs 30 Kg.

 a.  Is the order safe?

 b.  At what rate will you set the pump?

38.  Your patient is 48 cm tall and weighs 9.2 Kg. The medication is ordered at 125 mg/M². How much will the child receive?

39.  According to the literature, the safe range for the medication is 8 – 20 mg/Kg/day in four divided doses. What is the minimum safe dose per dose for your 18.3 Kg patient?

40.  D5NS is infusing into your patient at 45 ml/hr. She has an NG tube through which she has lost 180 ml in the previous shift. The doctor has ordered NS with 10 mEq KCl as replacement fluids. At what rate will the replacement fluids infuse?

41. Your 23.68 Kg patient has maintenance fluids ordered, to be given over the next 12 hours. At what rate will you set the pump?

42. The medication is available 0.75 mg/ml. The order is for 60 mcg/Kg for your 71.4 lb patient. How many ml will you give?

43. The literature gives a safe range of 20 – 50 mg/Kg/day in four divided doses. The doctor has ordered 100 mg every four hours. The child weighs 19 Kg. Is the doctor's order safe?

44. Your 27.3 Kg patient is put on half maintenance. At what rate will you set the IV pump to deliver the fluids?

45. Your patient has NS infusing at 30 ml/hr. The doctor orders a 500 ml bolus dose to infuse over the next four hours. The infusion rate will then revert to its pre-bolus rate. How much fluid will the patient receive over the next 24 hours?

46. The child is to receive 40 mcg/Kg/min. of the medication ordered. The medication is available 1 g in 250 ml. The patient weighs 29.8 Kg. How many mg will the patient receive per hour?

47. In the previous problem, at what rate would you set the pump for the calculated dose to infuse?

48. Your 73 lb patient has a medication ordered at 100 mg per dose. The safe range, per the pharmacy, is 10 – 25 mg/Kg/day in four divided doses. Is the doctor's order safe?

49. The medication is available at 125 mg/10 ml. The safe dose is 15 – 25 mg/Kg/day in three divided doses. Your patient weighs 22.7 Kg. The doctor has ordered 15 ml per dose. Is the order safe?

50. Available: 500 mg/10 ml in 10 ml vials
    Order: 175 mg in 50 ml of ½ NS

    a.  How much of the available medication should be added to the NS?

    b.  At what rate will you set the pump for this medication to infuse in 30 minutes?

    c.  The doctor has ordered the child should not receive IV fluid at more than 12 ml/hr/Kg. The child weighs 7.8 Kg. Will you need to call the doctor to question the order?

51. The doctor has ordered 150 mg of a medication three times daily for your pediatric patient, who weighs 27.8 Kg. The usual dose is 5 to 20 mg/Kg/day in divided doses. Is the doctor's order safe?

52. According to the literature, the medication's usual dose is 25 to 40 mg/Kg/day in divided doses. What is the safe range for your 29.6 lb patient?

53. The child is to receive a medication at 2.5 mcg/Kg/min. The child weighs 23.6 Kg. What is the hourly dosage in mg/hr?

54. Calculate the M$^2$ of a child weighing 11 lb 6 oz. and 23 in. long.

55. The recommended dose is 30 mg/M$^2$ to 50 mg/M$^2$. What is the safe range for your patient in problem 54?

56. The child has D5W NG replacement fluids ordered for the 146 ml of fluid lost to the NG in the prior shift. He is also to receive 1.5 maintenance fluid over the next 24 hours. The child weighs 22.46 Kg. What rate will you set for each fluid?

57. The order is for 450 mg of a medication every 8 hours. The safe dose per your reference is 60 – 90 mg/Kg/day. The drug is available 125 mg/ml. Your patient weighs 22.3 Kg.

    a.    What is the safe range for your patient?

    b.    Is the doctor's order safe?

    c.    How much of the medication will the child receive per dose in ml?

58. The doctor determines your pediatric patient is slightly dehydrated, and orders a 500 ml bolus of D5W to be infused over the next 8 hours. The child currently has D5W infusing at 40 ml/hr. What rate will you need to set for the next 8 hours to give the ordered bolus?

59. Your patient weighs 14.7 Kg. Your reference states the safe dose for a medication ordered is 40 to 70 mg/kg/day in four divided doses. The doctor has ordered 200 mg every four hours.

    a.    What is the safe range?

    b.    Is the doctor's order safe?

60. Calculate the M² for a pediatric patient who is 55 cm tall and weighs 13.7 Kg.

61. Using the M² calculated in problem 60, what is the safe dose for a medication to be given at 20 mg/M²?

62. A child is to receive 150 mg of a medication. The medication is available 750 mg of a powder in a 10 ml vial. You are to add enough fluid to the vial to create a 200 mg/ml concentration.

    a. How much fluid will you add to the vial to create the desired concentration?

    b. How much will you give your patient, in ml?

63. Your patient weighs 38.6 Kg. The doctor has ordered 1.5 x maintenance fluids per the usual 100-50-20 rule. How much IV fluid will your patient receive in the next 24 hours as maintenance fluids?

64. What is the M$^2$ for a newborn who weighs 8 lb 10 oz and is 22 inches long?

65. Your pediatric patient has an NG tube, with 78 ml of output in the past 12 hours. He has D5NS infusing at 40 ml/hr. The MD has ordered NG replacement fluids of D5NS with 10 mEq KCl. At what rate would you set the pump to replace the fluids lost through the NG tube?

66. The literature states the safe dosage range for the ordered medication is 40-70 mg/Kg/dose, not to exceed 6 g per day. Your patient weighs 37.2 Kg.

    a. What is the safe range for your patient?

    b. The doctor ordered 2 g every 8 hours. Is his order safe?

67. The doctor ordered the medication at 5 mg/Kg/day in four doses for your 42 Kg patient. The medication is available only in 10 ml vials containing 250 mg of the medication. How many ml will your patient receive per dose?

68. Calculate the safe dose for a 29.7 lb patient for a medication ordered at 7.5 mg/Kg/day.

69. The child is to get a bolus dose of 500 ml of D51/2 NS, infused over a four-hour period. At what rate will it infuse?

70. The neonate, who weighs 8 lb. 3 oz., is to receive 2x maintenance fluids. At what rate will they infuse over the next 24 hours?

71. The child has lost 130 ml through an NG tube. The fluid is to be replaced with D5NS during your 12-hour shift. The child currently has D5NS infusing at 45 ml/hr. At what rate will you set the pump to replace the lost fluid?

72. The doctor ordered ½ maintenance fluids for your 73-lb patient.

    a.   How much fluid will the patient receive in the next 24 hours?

    b.   At what infusion rate?

73. Calculate the $M^2$ for a patient 73 cm tall who weighs 25.4 Kg.

74. For the child whose $M^2$ you just calculated, for a medication ordered at 500 mg/$M^2$ per day in four divided doses, how much would the child receive per dose?

75. The usual dose of a medication, according to the literature, is 80-125 mg/Kg/day in three divided doses.

    a.   What is the safe range for your 82-lb patient?

    b.   The doctor has ordered 1 g of the medication every 6 hours. Is his order safe?

76. Calculate the M² for a patient who weighs 54.16 lb. and is 42.5 inches tall.

77. The doctor has ordered another medication for your patient in problem 76. His order reads "Give 400 mg/M²." What will your patient's dose be?

78. The doctor ordered maintenance fluids for your 107 lb patient. How much fluid will the patient receive in the next 24 hours, and at what rate will it infuse?

79. Calculate the M² for an adolescent patient who is 5 ft 7 in tall and weighs 163 lb.

80. The literature states the safe range for a medication is 30-50 mg/Kg/day in divided doses. The doctor has ordered 500 mg every 8 hours. The patient weighs 82 lb, and the medication comes in a 200 mg/5 ml concentration.

    a.  What is the safe range?

    b.    Is the doctor's order safe?

    c.    How much will the child receive per dose, in ml?

81.    The child is to get a 350 ml bolus of D5 1/2 NS over the next 5 hours. What will the hourly rate be?

82.    Calculate the safe dose for a medication ordered at 80 mg per $M^2$ for your patient, whose $M^2$ is 0.29.

83.    Your patient weighs 6.4 Kg and is 33 cm long. The order is for him to receive 0.38 mg/Kg/day, or 10 mg per $M^2$, with the dose not to exceed 2.5 mg per day. Calculate the daily dose both ways, based on the doctor's order.

84. Calculate the $M^2$ for a child who weighs 22 lb 9 oz and is 20 inches long.

85. The doctor ordered 75 mg/$M^2$ three times daily for the child in the previous problem. How much medication will the child receive in one day?

86. The child weighs 19.8 Kg, and the doctor orders 2 x maintenance fluids to be infused over the next 24 hours. At what rate will you set the pump?

87. Your patient has an NG tube, through which she has lost 173 ml in the past 12 hours. The doctor has ordered D5W with 10 mEq of KCl as replacement fluids. The patient currently has D5NS infusing. What rate will you set on the pump to infuse the NG replacement fluid?

88. The safe range for the ordered medication is 25 to 50 mg/Kg/day in divided doses. The doctor has ordered 100 mg every 6 hours for your 18.7 Kg patient. Is his order safe?

89. Your patient weighs 11.4 Kg. The literature states the usual dose of a medication is 20 mg/Kg. What is the safe dose for the medication?

90. Calculate the $M^2$ of a patient who is 117 cm tall and weighs 28.18 Kg.

91. For the child in the previous problem, what is the dosage range for a drug with a recommended dose of 5 to 15 mg/$M^2$?

92. The doctor has ordered a medication at 150 mg/$M^2$, or 10 mg/Kg/dose. Calculate your patient's dose both ways. The child's $M^2$ is 1.33, and she weighs 20 Kg.

93. The doctor has ordered a medication at 500 mg every 6 hours. Your reference states the safe dosage is 60 – 100 mg/Kg/day in divided doses. Your patient weighs 31.2 Kg. The medication is available in an oral form with a concentration of 25 mg/ml.

    a. Is the doctor's order safe?

b.    How much will the child get per day, in ml?

94.    The patient has NS infusing at 25 ml/hr. He has an NG tube, through which he has lost 200 ml during the shift prior to yours. The doctor has ordered replacement fluids of D5NS. At what rate should the replacement fluids infuse?

95.    The order is for a medication at 150 mg/$M^2$ for your patient, who has an $M^2$ of 0.57. How much should you give your patient, per the doctor's order?

96.    The safe range for the medication in the previous problem is 1.5 to 3.25 mg/Kg/day. Your patient weighs 25 Kg.

a.    What is the safe range for your patient?

b.    Based on this, was the doctor's order safe in problem 95?

97. The order is for 1.5 x maintenance fluids for your patient, who weighs 21.7 Kg. How much fluid will you give your patient in the next 24 hours, in compliance with the order?

98. The patient has lost 258 ml via NG tube in the previous 12 hour shift. IV fluids are D5 1/2 NS infusing at 45 ml/hr. Replacement fluids are D5 1/2 NS. At what rate will you set the pump to return the fluid lost to the NG over the next 12 hours?

99. The literature states the safe range of a medication is 75 – 125 mg/Kg/day in four divided doses. Your patient weighs 59 Kg. What is the safe per dose range for her?

100. Your patient weighs 13 lb 7 oz. The MD has ordered a medication at 28 mcg/Kg/min. The medication is available 150 mg in 100 ml. At what rate will you set the pump?

101. Your pediatric patient weighs 15.8 Kg. The antibiotic ordered has a concentration of 500 mg/20ml. The usual dose is 20 to 40 mg/Kg/day in three divided doses.

    a.    The doctor has ordered 300 mg/dose. Is this a safe dose?

    b.    The doctor changed the order to 100 mg/dose. Is this an accurate dose?

    c.    The doctor changes the order again, to 225 mg/dose. Is this dose accurate and safe?

102. The child weighs 47 pounds, and has a moderately severe infection. Kefzol has been ordered. For a moderately severe infection, Kefzol is to be given at 25 to 50 mg/Kg/day.

    a.    What is the safe range for this medication?

    b.    If the medication is given in 4 divided doses, what will the per dose range be?

    c.    The doctor has ordered 150 mg every 6 hours. Should you question the order?

103. Dopamine comes in 5 ml vials with a concentration of 200 mg/5 ml. The doctor's order is for "Dopamine 3 mcg/Kg/min IV. Dilute 100 mg dopamine in 100 ml D5 1/2 NS." The child weighs 16 pounds.

    a.    How many ml dopamine should be added to the 100 ml D5 1/2 NS to reach the ordered dilution?

    b.    How many mcg should the child receive per hour?

    c.    What would the flow rate be to infuse this dose?

104. Calculate the BSA ($M^2$) of a teenager who weighs 47.81 Kg and is 161.3 cm tall.

105. The recommended child's dose is 5 to 10 mg/$M^2$. Based on the $M^2$ you just calculated in problem 104, what is the recommended dose range for this teenager?

106. A cancer drug is ordered for a patient whose BSA is 1.31 $M^2$. The doctor orders 25 mg/$M^2$ IV. What dose will your patient receive?

107. A child weighing 17.63 Kg has an antibiotic ordered at 500 mg every 6 hours. The child's dosage in your reference for this medication is 80 – 200 mg/Kg/day in divided doses. The drug is available in a 250 mg/ml concentration.

   a.   How many mg will the child receive per day?

   b.   Is the drug dosage ordered per day within safe parameters?

   c.   How many ml will the child receive per dose?

108. Your patient weighs 18.62 Kg. The doctor has ordered the patient to receive 14 mg/hr of a medication which comes in a concentration of 2.8 mg/ml.

   a.   How many mcg/min/Kg will the patient receive?

   b.   At what rate will you set the pump to deliver this medication?

109. The doctor has ordered 1.5 x maintenance fluids for your pediatric patient, who weighs 24.77 Kg. How much fluid will your patient receive in the next 24 hours?

110. The doctor orders a medication at 3.5 mg/Kg/day, in three divided doses. Your patient weighs 36 pounds. The medication comes in 10 ml vials containing 100 mg of medication.

    a.    How many mg will the child receive per dose?

    b.    Per day?

    c.    How many ml per dose?

111. The order is for erythromycin 125 mg every 4 hours. The child weighs 29 lb. The desired range for this antibiotic is 30 – 50 mg/Kg/day in divided doses. The available medication comes 125 mg/5 ml.

    a.    Is the ordered dose safe?

    b.    How many ml will the child receive per dose, per the MD's order?

112. The doctor has ordered 80 mg of a medication every 8 hours. The child weighs 18.9 lb. Referenced dosage is 30 mg/Kg/day in divided doses. The medication is available in a concentration of 150 mg/5 ml.

    a.    Is the prescribed dose safe?

b.     How many ml should the child receive per dose, by the MD's order?

113.   The order is for digoxin 30 mcg every 12 hours. Your patient weighs 9.74 Kg. Your reference states a safe dosage is 0.006 – 0.012 mg/Kg/day. Available is digoxin 50 mcg/ml.

a.     Is the prescribed dose safe?

b.     How many ml a dose will the child receive?

114.   Your pediatric patient weighs 18.92 lb. The medication ordered has a concentration of 300 mg to 15 ml. The usual dose is 10 – 15 mg/Kg/day in two divided doses.

a.     The doctor ordered 150 mg a day, divided into two doses. Is this a safe dose?

b.     The doctor changed the order to 30 mg a dose with three doses a day. Is this safe?

c.     How much would you give in ml per dose for the doctor's 2nd order?

115. The doctor has ordered an antibiotic for your 24-lb. pediatric patient. The antibiotic is to be given at 20 – 40 mg/Kg/day.

    a.    What is the safe range for this antibiotic?

    b.    If the child is to get three doses per day, what is the per dose range?

116. Calculate the $M^2$ for a teenaged patient who is 5'2" tall and weighs 127 lb.

117. A medication has been ordered for a child which is to be given at 15 mg/$M^2$. Using the $M^2$ you just calculated in problem 116, what dose will the child receive?

118. The doctor ordered half maintenance fluids on your 34.52 Kg patient. What rate will you set on the pump to infuse these fluids in 12 hours?

119. Your pediatric patient has had abdominal surgery and now has an NG tube, which has suctioned 70 ml out in the past 12 hours. He has D5 1/2 NS with 20 mEq KCl infusing at 40 ml/hr. The doctor has ordered D5 1/2 NS with 20 mEq KCl for replacement of fluids lost via NG. To what rate should you reset the IV flow rate to follow the doctor's order?

120. A child who weighs 83 lb. is to receive a medication which has been ordered at 1 g every 8 hours. Your reference states that a child's safe dose for the medication is 75 to 125 mg/Kg/day in divided doses. The drug comes in a 100 mg/ml concentration.

    a.    How much (in mg) will the child receive per day, by the MD's order?

    b.    Is the doctor's order safe?

    c.    How many ml will the child receive per dose?

121. Calculate the $M^2$ for a child who weighs 14.75 Kg and is 43.6 cm tall.

122. The child is to receive 5 – 10 mg/M². Using the M² calculated in problem 121, what is the child's safe range of medication?

123. The doctor has ordered a medication at 7 mg/Kg/day in four divided doses. The patient weighs 44 lb. Your reference states the safe range is 30 – 40 mg every 8 hours.

   a.   How much will the child receive per dose under the doctor's order?

   b.   Is the doctor's order safe?

124. The medication is infusing at 23 ml/hr on a pump. The medicine is available 10 mg in 100 ml D5W. How many mcg/min/Kg is the patient receiving, for a 14.54 Kg patient?

125. The doctor has ordered IV fluids of D5 1/2 NS at 40 ml/hr for your post-op pediatric patient. The patient has an NG tube, which has drained 105 ml on the previous shift. NG replacement fluids ordered are D5NS with 20 mEq KCl. Determine how much you would give, and how you would set the pump or pumps.

126. A medication has been ordered 60 mcg/Kg/min for your pediatric patient. The medication comes in 25 ml vials containing 1 g of the medication. It is to be mixed to create a solution of 1000 mg in a 500 ml bag. The child weighs 30 Kg.

    a.    How many ml of the medication should be added to the 500 ml bag to get the ordered strength?

    b.    How many mg of the medication should the child receive per hour?

    c.    What flow rate should be set to infuse the medication per the doctor's order?

127. Your teen-aged patient has ovarian cancer. The initial round of the medication ordered is to be given at 260 mg/M$^2$/day in four divided doses for 21 days. The medication comes in 50 mg capsules. Your patient weighs 118 lb. and is 63 in. tall. How much should she receive per dose? How many capsules will this be per dose?

128. A medication is ordered at 70 mg every 6 hours for a 17 lb. 9 oz. child. The literature states safe dosage is 30 mg/Kg/day. The available medication: 500 mg in 250 ml of 0.45 NS.

    a.    What is the child's weight in Kg?

    b.     How many mg/day will the child receive by the doctor's order?

    c.     Is the doctor's order safe, by the literature?

    d.     What will be the ml per dose, by the doctor's order?

129. A 54-pound child has an order for 250 mg of an antibiotic four times daily. The antibiotic come at 100 mg/5 ml, with the usual dose 15 – 40 mg/Kg/day in three divided doses.

    a.     What is the per dose range, according to the literature?

    b.     Is the doctor's order safe?

    c.     How many ml should the child receive per dose, following the MD's order?

130. Your fragile 13-month-old HIV-positive patient has developed a herpes simplex infection. The doctor has ordered acyclovir sodium 30 mg/Kg/day in three divided doses. The child weighs 26 pounds and is 28 inches long.

    a.     What is her $M^2$?

b. The label reads 750 mg/M² per day for 7 days. What is the per dose and per day safe dose for this child?

c. Is the doctor's order safe?

131. Your patient weighs 17 Kg and is 82 cm tall. What is his M²?

132. Your patient is to receive 2 – 5 mg/M² of a medication. Based on the M² you calculated in the previous problem, what is the safe dose range?

133. A child weighing 8 lb 7 oz is to receive a medication at 6 mcg/Kg/min. The medication is available 100 mg in 100 ml. At what rate would you set a pump to infuse the correct amount?

134. The child weighs 44 lb. The medication's safe dose is 15 to 25 mg/Kg/day in four divided doses. The doctor has ordered 100 mg/dose. Is his order safe?

135. A child has been admitted. The child is 3'8" tall and weighs 55 lb. Her medication has been ordered at 14 mg/M$^2$ per dose. How much will you give per dose?

136. The child has an NG tube which has drained 135 ml in the past 12 hours. IV fluids are ½ NS at 40 ml/hr. Replacement fluids ordered are ½ NS with 20 mEq potassium. At what rate will you set the pump to replace the fluid lost to the NG tube?

137. Your pediatric patient has an antibiotic ordered which is available at 300 mg/10 ml in a suspension. The patient weighs 16.9 Kg. The usual order is 20 – 30 mg/Kg/day in three divided doses. The doctor has ordered 250 mg/dose. Is this dose safe?

**Questions 138 – 140 are related**

138. The medication is available in a concentration of 100 mg/5 ml in 10 ml vials. The directions indicate you are to dilute 30 mg of the medication in 50 ml of D5W. How much of the medication should be added to the 50 ml of D5W to get the desired dilution?

139. Your 15.4 Kg patient is to receive 8 mcg/Kg/min of the above medication. How much will they receive per hour?

140. What flow rate would you set to infuse this dose?

141. The doctor has ordered 70 mg of a medication every 12 hours. The child weighs 11 lb 5 oz. The drug dosage for the medication in the literature is 25 mg/Kg/day in divided doses. Is the dose the doctor ordered safe?

142. What is the M² of a patient weighing 48.7 Kg who is 142.8 cm tall?

143. The doctor has ordered 1.5 x maintenance fluids for your 29.54 Kg patient. At what rate will you set the pump to infuse these fluids over the next 24 hours?

144. The child has ½ maintenance fluids ordered. He weighs 11.1 Kg. How much should he get in the next 24 hours? What flow rate would you set to deliver this?

145. What is the $M^2$ of a patient who is 4'7" tall and weighs 68 lb?

146. The doctor has ordered a 500 ml bolus dose of D5 1/2 NS for your pediatric patient, who currently has D5 1/2 NS infusing at 35 ml/hr. At what rate will you set the pump to infuse the bolus dose over the next four hours?

147. Your patient is 50 inches tall. She weighs 78 lb. She is to receive 24 mg/$M^2$ per dose of an ordered medication. How much will you give?

148. The five-year-old patient, who weighs 52 lb, has a severe ear infection, and the doctor has prescribed amoxicillin in a liquid form with a concentration of 125 mg in 5 ml. The usual dose is 20 – 40 mg/Kg/day in three divided doses. The doctor has ordered 300 mg every 6 hours.

    a.    What is the safe range?

    b.    Is the doctor's order safe?

149. The 8-year-old post-op patient has received an accidental narcotic overdose, and is now unresponsive. The doctor orders 0.5 ml Narcan to counteract the narcotic. The child weighs 66 pounds. Safe dose is 0.005 to 0.01 mg/Kg, and the Narcan is available 400 mcg/ml. What is the safe range, and is the doctor's order safe?

150. Your pediatric cancer patient is to receive doxorubicin 30 mg a week. The child is 42 inches tall and weighs 57 lb. The medication is available 25 mg in 50 ml of D5W. Safe dose is 20 – 30 mg/M$^2$ once a week.

    a.    What is the child's M$^2$?

    b.    What is the safe range for the medication for this child?

c.    Is the doctor's order safe?

d.    How many ml will the child receive per dose by the doctor's order?

# ANSWERS

# FUNDAMENTAL DOSAGE CALCULATIONS

## Playing with conversions:

1.    90 ml = _____ Tbsp = _____ tsp

    Tbsp = 1 Tbsp/15 ml x 90 ml = **6 Tbsp**

    Tsp = 1 tsp/5 ml x 90 ml = **18 tsp OR** 3 tsp/1 Tbsp x 6 Tbsp = 18 tsp


2.    720 ml = _____ pints = _____ cups = _____ oz.

    pt = 1 pt/480 ml x 720 ml = **1.5 pt**
    c = 2 c/1 pt x 1.5 pt = **3 c OR** c = 1 c/240 ml x 720 ml = 3 c
    oz = 1 oz/30 ml x 720 ml = **24 oz**

3.    How many drops in one cup?

    gtt = 15 gtt/1 ml x 240 ml/1 c x 1 c = **3600 gtt**


4.    How many tsp in 1 pt?

    tsp = 1 tsp/5 ml x 480 ml/1 pt x 1 pt = **96 tsp**


5.    In lb, how much does a 45 Kg patient weigh?

    lb = 2.2 lb/1 Kg x 45 Kg = **99 lb**

6.  a.  Your patient weighed 54 Kg and was told to lose 10% of his body weight. He did so. How much did he lose, in lb?

    lb = 2.2 lb/1 Kg x 5.4 Kg = **11.9 lb**

    b.  Your patient weighed 300 lb and was told to lose 10% of his body weight. He did so. How much does he weigh now, in Kg?

    300 lb – 30 lb = 270 lb Kg = 1 Kg/2.2 lb x 270 lb = **122.7 Kg**

7.  150 mg = _____ gr

    gr = 1 gr/60 mg x 150 mg = **2.5 gr**

8.  3.5 pt = _____ ml

    ml = 480 ml/1 pt x 3.5 pt = **1680 ml**

9.  3000 mcg = _____ mg = _____ g

    mg = 1 mg/1000 mcg x 3000 mcg = **3 mg**
    g = 1 g/1000 mg x 3 mg = **0.003 g**

10. 14 oz = _____ ml

    ml = 30 ml/1 oz x 14 oz = **420 ml**

11. The order is for 2 tsp of cough syrup every 4 hours. Available: 10 mg/ml

    a.  How many gtt will the patient get per dose?
        gtt = 15 gtt/ml x 5 ml/tsp x 2 tsp = **150 gtt**

    b.  How many mg will the patient get per dose?
        mg = 10 mg/ml x 10 ml = **100 mg**

**And now, some regular fundamentals math problems**

11.  Order: 60 mg codeine PO
     Available: codeine gr ½ per tab
     How many tabs should you give?

     tabs = 1 tab/0.5 gr x 1 gr/60 mg x 60 mg/d.o. = **2 tabs**

12.  Order: Reglan 20 mg
     Available: Reglan 10 mg/ml

     How many ml should you give?

     ml = 1 ml/10 mg x 20 mg = **2 ml**

13.  Order: Nembutal gr v PO [grains may be given in Roman numerals]
     Available: Nembutal 100 mg capsules
     How many caps will you give?

     caps = 1 cap/100 mg x 60 mg/1 gr x 5 gr/d.o. = 300/100 = **3 caps**

14.  Order: oxycodone 50 mg PO
     Available: oxycodone oral solution 20 mg/ml
     How much will you give?

     ml = 1 ml/20 mg x 50 mg = **2.5 ml**

15.  Order: ethambutol 15 mg/kg/24 hours PO to an adult weighing 176 lb.
     Label: ethambutol 400 mg/tab
     How many tabs should you give?

     mg = 15 mg/Kg x 1 Kg/2.2 lb x 176 lb = 2640/2.2 = 1200 mg
     tabs = 1 tab/400 mg x 1200 mg = **3 tabs**

16. Doctor's order: tetracycline 350 mg PO
Available: tetracycline suspension 125 mg/ml
How much will you give?

ml = 1 ml/125 mg x 350 mg = **2.8 ml**

17. Order: levothyroxine 0.075 mg PO daily
Available: levothyroxine 50 mcg/tab
How many tabs will you give?

tab = 1 tab/50 mcg x 1000 mcg/1 mg x 0.075 mg = **1.5 tabs**

18. The medication comes as 500 mg in a powdered form, to which you are to add 75 ml of sterile water. The doctor's order is for 400 mg one-time PO dose. How much will you give?

ml = 75 ml/500 mg x 400 mg = 30,000/500 = **60 ml**

19. Phenergan 75 mg PO ordered
Phenergan syrup 25 mg/5 ml available
How many tsp should you give? (Note: here you must start with a conversion factor.)

tsp = 1 tsp/5 ml x 5 ml/25 mg x 75 mg = 375/125 = **3 tsp**

20. Order: Nembutal sodium gr 1.5 PO
Label: Nembutal sodium 100 mg/cap
How many caps should you give?

mg = 60 mg/gr x 1.5 gr = 90 mg
caps = 1 cap/100 mg x 90 mg = 90/100 so give **1 cap**

**Remember: up to a 10% difference between what is ordered and what is given is still OK.**

21. Order: PCN 800,000 units IM
Available: PCN 1,000,000 units per ml
How much will you give the patient?

ml = 1 ml/1,000,000 units x 800,000 units = **0.8 ml**

**Note: If your answer is a decimal less than 1, you must put a zero before the decimal.**

22. Order: 30 mg Nitro-Dur transdermally, change every 6 hours.
Available: 1 in = 15 mg (Note: Nitro-Dur is a paste)

    a.    How much will you give per dose?
           inches = 1 in/15 mg x 30 mg = **2 in**

    b.    How much will you give per day?
           in = 2 in/dose x 4 doses = **8 in**

23. Order: dilute the medication with 80 ml of NS, and give a 20 mg IV dose.
Available: vial of medication containing 200 mg in 2 ml, which you are to dilute.
How much will you give?

ml = 82 ml/200 mg x 20 mg = **8.2 ml**

24. Lovenox 1 mg/kg SQ has been ordered. It is available in a preloaded syringe of 80
mg/0.8 ml. Your patient weighs 165 lb. How many mg will you give? How many ml?

mg ordered = 1 mg/Kg x 1 Kg/2.2 lb x 165 lb = **75 mg**
ml = 0.8 ml/80 mg x 75 mg = 60/80 = 0.75 = **0.8 ml** rounded

25. A COPD patient comes in in respiratory distress, and the ER physician orders
Solumedrol 60 mg IV push. The drug is available as 125 mg in 2 ml. How many ml will
you give?

ml = 2 ml/125 mg x 60 mg = 0.96 = **1 ml**

26.  Order: Clindamycin 225 mg IM every 6 hr for 7 days
     Available: Clindamycin 75 mg/ml in a 5 ml vial

   a.  How much will you give with each dose?
       ml = 1 ml/75 mg x 225 mg = **3 ml**

   b.  What is the total dosage the doctor has ordered, in mg?
       ml = 3 ml/dose x 4 doses/day x 7 days = 84 ml
       mg = 75 mg/ml x 84 ml = **6300 mg**

27.  Valproic acid is ordered 15 mg/kg/day. It is available as 250 mg caps. Your patient weighs 73 pounds. How much will he get per day in mg? How many capsules?

   mg = 15 mg/Kg x 1 Kg/2.2 lb x 73 lb = 1095/2.2 = 497.7 mg
   caps = 1 cap/250 mg x 497.7 mg = **2 caps**

28.  The patient is to receive 240 ml via feeding tube. You start the feeding at 0700 at 20 ml/hr, and have instructions to increase the rate every hour, by 10 ml/hr to a maximum of 50 ml/hr. At what time will the bag be empty?

|  |  |  |
|---|---|---|
|  |  | 240 ml |
|  | 0700-0800 | −20 |
|  |  | 220 ml |
| Empty at **1300** | 0800-0900 | −30 |
|  |  | 190 ml |
|  | 0900-1000 | −40 |
|  |  | 150 ml |
|  | 1000-1300 | −150 none left |

29.  The medication is a powder, 500 mg per vial. You are to add enough fluid to create a 40 mg/ml concentration. How much fluid will you add?

   ml = 1 ml/40 mg x 500 mg = **12.5 ml**

30. Your patient weighs 44 pounds. You are to give 0.5 mg/kg of a medication, per dose. The medication comes in a concentration of 5 mg/ml. How much will you give?

ml = 1 ml/5 mg x 0.5 mg/Kg x 1 Kg/2.2 lb x 44 lb = 22/11 = **2 ml**

31. The doctor has ordered iii grains of phenobarbital every eight hours. The medication comes in 2 ml vials containing 65 mg/ml. How much will you give per dose?

ml = 1 ml/65 mg x 60 mg/1 gr x 3 gr = 180/65 = **2.8 ml**

32. The oral solution ordered is available 2 g in 100 ml. The doctor's order is for 300 mg. How much will you give in ml?

ml = 100 ml/2000 mg x 300 mg = 30,000/2000 = **15 ml**

33. The doctor's order reads digoxin 375 mcg daily. The tablets available are 0.125 mg. How many tablets should you give?

tabs = 1 tab/0.125 mg x 1 mg/1000 mcg x 375 mcg = **3 tabs**

34. Your patient is to get 12 mEq of potassium every 6 hours. The potassium available comes 40 mEq per packet, to be dissolved in 30 ml of juice. How much should you give per dose?

ml = 30 ml/40mEq x 12 mEq = **9 ml**

35. The order is for 8 mg of methadone. Methadone is available in a 10 ml vial, with a concentration of 5 mg/ml. How much will you give?

ml = 1 ml/5 mg x 8 mg = **1.6 ml**

36. Ordered: 1/120 gr digoxin (Change fractions to decimals; don't round till the answer)
    Available: 0.25 mg tablets
    How many tablets will you give?

    tabs = 1 tab/0.25 mg x 50 mg/1 gr x 0.00833 gr = 0.4998/0.25 = **2 tabs**

37. Your patient is to get 800,000 units of penicillin.
    The penicillin available comes 200,000 units/ml in a 10 ml vial. How much will you give?

    ml = 1 ml/200,000 units x 800,000 units = **4 ml**

38. Aspirin is available in 10 gr tablets. The doctor's order is for 1200 mg every four hours. How many tabs will you give per dose?

    tabs = 1 tab/10 gr x 1 gr/60 mg x 1200 mg = **2 tabs**

39. An antibiotic has been ordered, 0.2 g four times daily. The available medication is 100 mg per capsule. How many capsules will you give per day?

    caps = 1 cap/100 mg x 200 mg/dose x 4 doses = **8 caps**

40. Robinul comes in a 5 ml vial containing 0.2 mg/ml. The doctor has ordered 0.4 mg every four hours as needed for congestion. Your patient requires four doses in a 24-hour period. How much was that in ml?

    ml = 1 ml/0.2 mg x 0.4 mg/dose x 4 doses = 1.6/0.2 = **8 ml**

41. Tube feeding is to give 400 ml starting at 0700. You are to start it at 20 ml/hr, increasing by 20 ml/hr every 2 hours to a maximum of 80 ml/hr. (a) At what time would that rate be reached? (b) When would the bag be empty?

Hits 80 ml/hr at **1300**
Bag empty at **1500**

|  |  |
|---|---|
|  | 400 ml |
| 0700-0900 20/ml/hr | – 40 ml |
|  | 360 ml |
| 0900 – 1100 40 ml/hr | – 80 ml |
|  | 280 ml |
| 1100 – 1300 60 ml/hr | –120 ml |
|  | 160 ml |
| 1300-1500 80 ml/hr | –160 ml |
|  | 0 ml |

42. The order is for phenobarbital 70 mg twice a day; available is phenobarbital 65 mg/1 ml. How much will you give per dose? Per day?

ml = 1 ml/65 mg x 70 mg = **1.1 ml/dose**
ml = 1.1 ml/dose x 2 doses = **2.2 ml/day**

43. You are to give 1800 units of a medication. The available dose strength is 1000 units per 1.5 ml. How much will you give?

ml = 1.5 ml/1000 units x 1800 units = 2700/1000 = **2.7 ml**

44. The doctor's order is for 5 mg of Lasix. The pharmacy has it available in a 2 ml vial, 10 mg per ml. How much should you give?

ml = 1 ml/10 mg x 5 mg = **0.5 ml**

45. Order: 260 mcg Robinul. Available: Robinul 0.2 mg/ml in a 10 ml vial. Your patient should receive how much?

ml = 1 ml/0.2 mg x 1 mg/1000 mcg x 260 mcg = **1.3 ml**

46. The available medication comes 1200 mg in a 2.5 ml vial. The doctor has ordered 800 mg. Calculate the patient's dose.

    ml = 2.5 ml/1200 mg x 800 mg = **1.7 ml**

47. Order: 170 mg of a medication. It is available in a liquid form, 100 mg/ml. Dose:

    ml = 1 ml/100 mg x 170 mg = **1.7 ml**

48. A medication which comes 1.5 mg in 2 ml is to be used to prepare a 0.75 mg dosage for your patient. How much fluid will be required in order to accurately mix the correct dose?

    ml = 2 ml/1.5 mg x 0.75 mg = **1 ml**

49. You are to add 600 mg of a medication to an IV bag (although normally the pharmacy does this). The solution available to use comes 500 mg in 10 ml. How much will you add?

    ml = 10 ml/500 mg x 600 mg = **12 ml**

50. You are to prepare a 0.6 g dose from a 300 mg per 2 ml solution. How much will you need?

    ml = 2 ml/300 mg x 600 mg = **4 ml**

51. You are to add enough fluid to a 75 mg vial to create a 30mg/ml concentration, then give a 22 mg dose. How much fluid should you add, and how much (in ml) will you give?

    ml = 1 ml/30 mg x 75 mg = **2.5 ml to add**
    ml = 1 ml/30 mg x 22 mg = **0.7 ml to give**

52. The order is for 2 tsp of cough syrup every 4 hours. Available: 10 mg/ml.

   a. How many gtt will the patient get per dose?
   gtt = 15 gtt/ml x 5 ml/tsp x 2 tsp = **150 gtt**

   b. How many mg will the patient get per dose?
   mg = 10 mg/ml x 5 ml/tsp x 2 tsp = **100 mg**

53. The order is for Equamil 0.2 g by mouth every 4 hours.
   Available: Equamil 400 mg per tab

   a. How many mg would you give per dose?
   mg = 1000 mg/1 g x 0.2 g = **200 mg**

   b. How many tabs would this be?
   tab = 1 tab/400 mg x 200 mg = **0.5 tab**

   c. How many tabs would you give in 48 hours?
   tabs = 0.5 tab/4 hr x 48 hr = **6 tabs**

54. Order: 0.6 g of a medication PO every 6 hours
   Available: 200 mg/5 ml
   Give: _____ ml in 24 hours

   ml = 5 ml/200 mg x 1000 mg/1 g x 0.6 g = 15 ml/dose
   15 ml/6 hours x 24 hours **= 60 ml in 24 hours**

55. You have reconstituted a medicine, creating a strength of 100 mg/ml. The order is to give 0.3 g every 8 hours. Total dose in 3 days? (Remember, you can only give medicine in the form it comes in, which here is a liquid, so you are looking for ml.)

   ml = 1 ml/100 mg x 1000 mg/1 g x 0.3 g/8 hr x 24 hr/1 day x 3 days = **27 ml**

56. At 0800 you begin a G-tube feeding of 930 ml, starting at 30 ml/hr. The MD's orders say to increase the rate hourly by 10 ml/hr to a maximum of 80 ml/hr.

|  |  |
|---|---|
|  | 930 ml |
| 0800-0900 | - 30 ml |
|  | 900 ml |
| 0900-1000 | - 40 ml |
|  | 860 ml |
| 1000-1100 | -50 ml |
|  | 810 ml |
| 1100-1200 | - 60 ml |
|  | 750 ml |
| 1200-1300 | -70 ml |
|  | 680 ml |
| 1300-2100 | -640 ml 8 hr @ 80 |
|  | 40 ml |
| 2100-2130 | -40 ml |
|  | 0 ml |

a. At what time will the rate reach 80 ml/hr?
Will reach 80 ml/hr at **1300**

b. At what time will the bag be empty?
Bag will be empty at **2130**

57. The patient is to get 30 mg/Kg/day of a medication in three divided doses. He weighs 187 lb. The medication is available 100 mg/ml.

a. mg per dose?
$$mg = \frac{30 \text{ mg/Kg}}{\text{per day}} \times 1 \text{ Kg}/2.2 \text{ lb} \times 187 \text{ lb} = 2550 \text{ mg/day} \times 1 \text{ day}/3 \text{ doses} = 850 \text{ mg per dose}$$

b. ml per day?
ml = 1 ml/100 mg x 2550 mg = **25.5 ml**

58. Order: 1.5 mg/Kg/day for a patient who weighs 92.6 Kg
Available: 125 mg/ml

a. How many ml/day will the patient receive? (Carry answer to hundredths)
ml/day = 1 ml/125 mg x 1.5 mg/Kg x 92.6 Kg = **1.11 ml**
per day

b.  How many mg will he receive in 48 hours?
    mg = 125 mg/ml x 1.11 ml/day x 2 days = **277.5 mg** (less due to rounding)
    **OR** mg = 1.5 mg/Kg/day x 92.6 Kg = 138.9 mg/day x 2 days = 277.8 mg

59. Order: gr iii phenobarbital every 6 hours prn agitation
    Available: 60 mg tablets
    How many tablets will you give per dose?

    tabs = 1 tab/60 mg x 60 mg/1 gr x 3 gr = **3 tabs**

60. The patient is to receive 0.2 units/Kg of insulin. The patient weighs 320 lb. The insulin is available 100 units/ml.

    a.  How many units will the patient receive? (Remember, for units you must round to the nearest whole number.)
        units = 0.2 units/Kg x 1 Kg/2.2 lb x 320 lb = 29.09 = **29 units**

    b.  How many ml will that be? (Round to nearest tenth.)
        ml = 1 ml/100 units x 29 units = 0.29 = **0.3 ml**

61. The doctor has ordered 60 mg of Phenergan. It is available 20 mg/5 ml. How many tsp should you give?

    tsp = 1 tsp/5 ml x 5 ml/20 mg x 60 mg = **3 tsp**

62. Clindamycin has been ordered 250 mg IM every 6 hours for 7 days. It is available 50 mg/ml in a 5 ml vial. How much will you need (in mg) for the 7-day supply? How many vials would that be?

    mg = 250 mg/6 hr x 24 hr/1 day x 7 days = **7000 mg**
    vials = 1 vial/5 ml x 1 ml/50 mg x 7000 mg = **28 vials**

63. You are to add 700 mg of a medication to an IV bag. The solution available comes 250 mg in 5 ml. How much will you add?

    ml = 5 ml/250 mg x 700 mg = **14 ml**

64. The order is for Procan 500 mg loading dose (a large initial dose, intended to begin setting up a given level in the patient's bloodstream), followed by 250 mg every 3 hours. Available: Procan 100 mg tabs.

    a.    How many tabs will you give as a loading dose?
        tabs = 1 tab/100 mg x 500 mg = **5 tabs**

    b.    How many tabs will you give for each dose after the loading dose?
        tabs = 1 tab/100 mg x 250 mg = **2.5 tabs**

    c.    After the loading dose is given, how many additional tabs will you need for the next 24 hours?
        tabs = 2.5 tabs/3 hr x 24 hr = **20 tabs**

65. The order is for metronidazole 3 g per day in 4 equal divided doses. The medicine is available as 500 mg tabs. How many tabs will you give with each dose?

    tab/dose = 1 tab/500 mg x 1000 mg/1 g x 3 g/day x 1 day/4 doses = **1.5 tab/dose**

66. Glycopyrrolate 0.1 mg is ordered. Glycopyrrolate is available in 10 ml vials with a concentration of 0.2 mg/ml. How many ml will you give your patient?

    ml = 1 ml/0.2 mg x 0.1 mg = **0.5 ml**

67. You are to give your patient 750 mg of a medication available 0.3 g in 1 ml. How much will you give?

    ml = 1 ml/300 mg x 750 mg = **2.5 ml**

68. Cefotaxime comes in 50 ml vials with a concentration of 300 mg/ml. The doctor's order is for 60 mg/Kg/dose, with one dose every 6 hours. The patient weighs 30 Kg.

    a.    How much will you give per dose?
        ml = 1 ml/300 mg x 60 mg/Kg x 30 Kg = **6 ml**

b.  How much will you give per day?
ml = 6 ml/dose x 4 doses/day = **24 ml**
**OR** ml = 6 ml/6 hours x 24 hours/day = 24 ml

69. You are to reconstitute a vial of 50,000 units of urokinase to a concentration of 2000 units per ml. How much diluent will you use?

ml = 1 ml/2000 units x 50,000 units = **25 ml**

70. Available scored tablets come in three sizes: 10, 20, and 40 gr. The doctor has ordered 1200 mg of the medication. How many tablets would you give of each strength to follow the doctor's order? (Solve the problems using the fewest number of tablets possible, and without cutting any tablets.)

a.  10 gr    mg = 60 mg/gr x 10 gr = 600 mg ; 1200 mg/600 mg = **2 tabs**

b.  20 gr    mg = 60 mg/gr x 20 gr = 1200 mg; 1200/1200 = **1 tab**

c.  40 gr    mg = 60 mg/gr x 40 gr = 2400 mg; 1200/2400 = **0.5 tab**

71. Order: Nembutal gr iii PO
Available: Nembutal 90 mg capsules
How many capsules will you give?

caps = 1 cap/90 mg x 60 mg/1 gr x 3 gr = **2 caps**

72. The doctor has ordered gr ii of phenobarbital for the agitated patient. The medication is available in 2 ml vials containing 130 mg/ml of phenobarbital. How much will you give your patient?

ml = 1 ml/130 mg x 60 mg/1 gr x 2 gr = **0.9 ml**

73. The order is for 1/120 gr of a medication which is available in 0.25, 0.5, and 1 mg tablets. Which will you give? (Give fewest tabs possible.)

MD ordered 60 mg/1 gr x 0.00833 gr = 0.499998 mg = 0.5 mg, so **give one 0.5 mg tab**

74. Your patient weighs 66 pounds. You are to give 0.5 mg/Kg of a medication per dose, twice a day. The medication comes in a concentration of 5 mg/ml. How much will you give per day?

ml = 1 ml/5 mg x 0.5 mg/Kg x 30 Kg = 3 ml/dose
    per dose
3 ml/dose x 2 doses/day = **6 ml/day**

75. Your patient is to get 8 mEq of potassium every 4 hours. The potassium available comes 40 mEq per packet, to be dissolved in 30 ml of juice. How much should you give per dose?

ml = 30 ml/40 mEq x 8 mEq = **6 ml**

76. An antibiotic has been ordered 0.4 g six times daily. Available are 200 mg capsules of the antibiotic. How many capsules will you give per day?

caps = 1 cap/200 mg x 1000 mg/g x 0.4 g/dose x 6 doses/day = **12 caps**

77. The doctor has ordered 1/120 gr digoxin. The pharmacy has 0.25 mg tablets. How many tablets should you give to obey the MD's order?

tabs = 1 tab/0.25 mg x 60 mg/1 gr x 0.00833 gr = **2 tabs**

78. The doctor has ordered cefoxitin 75 mg/Kg/day, in 6 equal doses (that is, a dose every 4 hours). The medicine is available 1.5 g in 100 ml of D5W. The patient weighs 88 pounds.

    a.   How much is the patient receiving per day, in mg?

        mg = 75 mg/Kg x 40 Kg = **3000 mg per day**

    b.   How much should you give per dose in ml?

        ml = 100 ml/1500 mg x 3000 mg/day x 1 day/6 doses = **33.3 ml**

79. Flecainide, an antiarrhythmic, is available in 50, 100, and 150 mg scored tablets. Which tablets will you choose for a 500 mg daily dose, and how many tablets will you give? (The rules: use the fewest number of tabs possible. Do not cut tabs if you can give the dose without doing so. You can give more than one size tab in a single dose.)

| 2 | 150 mg tabs | = | 300 mg | **OR** | 3 | 150 mg tabs | = | 450 mg |
| 2 | 100 mg tabs | = | 200 mg | | 1 | 50 mg tab | = | 50 mg |
| | | | 500 mg | | | | | 500 mg |

80. The doctor orders 35 mEq of potassium for your hypokalemic patient. The medication comes in 10 or 20 mEq capsules, so you can't use either of those, since capsules can't be split. An oral solution with 20 mEq in 15 ml is available. How much will you give? (Round to the nearest 100$^{th}$.)

ml = 15 ml/20 mEq x 35 mEq = **26.25 ml**

81. The MD has ordered a medication with dose based on the size of the patient. The patient is to get 5 mg/Kg of the medication. The patient weighs 209 pounds.

a. How many mg of medicine will he receive?

mg = 5 mg/Kg x 95 Kg = **475 mg**

b. If the medication is available 50 mg/ml, how many ml should you give the patient?

ml = 1 ml/50 mg x 475 mg = **9.5 ml**

82. PCN G comes in a vial containing 10,000,000 units. You are to reconstitute it to a concentration of 400,000 units/ml. How much diluent must you add to the vial?

ml = 1 ml/400,000 units x 10,000,000 units = **25 ml**

83. The medication prescribed is available 50 mg in 200 ml. The doctor has ordered 30 mg per day in three divided doses. How much should you give per dose?

ml = 200 ml/50 mg x 30 mg/day x 1 day/3 doses = **40 ml**

84.  The order is for levofloxacin by mouth, with an initial (first) order of 400 mg, followed by 250 mg three times daily thereafter. Only 100 mg tablets are available.

    a.    How many tablets will be in the initial dose?

        tab = 1 tab/100 mg x 400 mg = **4 tabs**

    b.    How many tablets will be in each subsequent dose?

        tab = 1 tab/100 mg x 250 mg = 2.**5 tabs**

85.  The doctor has ordered a loading dose of 450 mg of a medication, followed by a 300 mg dose every 6 hours for one week. The medication comes in 150 mg tablets. Not counting the loading dose (so the clock starts six hours after the loading dose), how many tablets will be needed for one week?

    tabs = 1 tab/150 mg x 300 mg/6 hr x 24 hr/1 day x 7 days = **56 tabs**

86.  The patient is having chest pain, so the doctor orders nitroglycerin paste 30 mg every 6 hours. The medication comes as a paste in small packets containing 15 mg = 1 inch. How many packets will be required for one day?

    inches = 1 in/15 mg x 30 mg/6 hr x 24 hr/1 day = 8 inches
    packets = 1 packet/1 in x 8 in = **8 packets**

87.  The medication is to be given at 3 mg/Kg/dose to a patient weighing 242 pounds. The medication is available 100 mg/ml. How much will you give per dose, in ml?

    ml = 1 ml/100 mg x 3 mg/Kg x 110 Kg = **3.3 ml**

88. The patient is to be fed via G tube. The MD orders a 300 ml initial feeding to test the patient's tolerance, starting at 30 ml/hr and increasing by 10 ml/hr every 2 hours to a maximum of 60 ml/hr. At what time will you set the rate at 60 ml/hr, assuming you start the feeding at 1800?

**At midnight (2400), rate will increase to 60 ml/hr**

300 ml
-60 ml 30 ml/hr x 2 hr 1800-2000
240 ml
-80 ml 40 ml/hr x 2 hr 2000-2200
160 ml
-100 ml 50 ml/hr x 2 hr 2000-2400
60 ml

89. The doctor has ordered 4 grains per day of a medication which is available only in 30 mg tablets. The ordered reads "4 gr in 4 divided doses." How many tablets will the patient receive per dose?

tabs/dose = 1 tab/30 mg x 60 mg/1 gr x 4 gr/day x 1 day/4 doses = **2 tabs**

90. Your patient is to receive 640 ml of fluid through a G tube. You start the feeding at 20 ml/hr at 0700, and orders are to increase it by 20 ml/hr every two hours to a maximum of 80 ml/hr. At what time will the bag be empty?

**At 1800, the bag will be empty.**

640 ml
-40 ml 20 ml/hr x 2 hr 0700-0900
600 ml
-80 ml 40 ml/hr x 2 hr 0900-1100
520 ml
-120 ml 60 ml/hr x 2 hr 1100-1300
400 ml
-400 ml 80 ml/hr x 5 hr 1300-1800
0

91. Order: 1/150 gr of a medication
Available: 0.2 mg tablets
How many tablets will you give per dose?

tabs = 1 tab/0.2 mg x 60 mg/1 gr x 0.00667 gr = **2 tab**

92. Your patient is to receive 50 mg of a medication which comes 5 mg/ml. How many tsp will she get?

   tsp = 1 tsp/5 ml x 1 ml/5 mg x 50 mg/d.o. = 50/25 = **2 tsp**


93. The medication is available 250 mg in 2 ml NS. The doctor has ordered 700 mg. How much will the patient receive?

   ml = 2 ml/250 mg x 700 mg/d.o. = **5.6 ml**


94. The patient's order is for 15 mcg per Kg. The medication is available 1 mg/ml. How much will the patient receive if he weighs 115 Kg?

   ml = 1 ml/mg x 1 mg/1000mcg x 15 mcg/Kg x 115 Kg = **1.7 ml**


95. You are to reconstitute a powdered medication which comes 500 mg in a 10 ml vial. You add 8 ml of sterile water to the vial. The doctor's order is for 275 mg. How much will that be in ml?

   ml = 8 ml/500 mg x 275 mg/d.o. = **4.4 ml**


96. The doctor has ordered v grains of a medication which is available only in 300 mg tablets. How many tablets will you give?

   tab = 1 tab/300 mg x 60 mg/1 gr x 5 gr/d.o. = **1 tab**


97. The medication was ordered as an oral solution containing 10 mg/ml. The doctor has ordered a 250 mg dose every 6 hours. How much will the patient receive in one day?

   ml = 1 ml/10 mg x 250 mg/6 hours x 24 hours/1 day = **100 ml a day**

98. The doctor has ordered the patient to receive feedings through a G tube. He has ordered the feedings be started at 20 ml/hr, then increased by 20 ml/hr every two hours until the patient is receiving 100 ml/hr. You hang a 500 ml bag at 0900. At what time will the bag be empty?

| | | | | |
|---|---|---|---|---|
| | | | 500 ml | |
| 0900 – 1100 | 20 ml/hr x 2 hrs | = | - 40 ml | |
| | | | 460 ml | |
| 1100 – 1300 | 40 ml/hr x 2 hrs | = | - 80 ml | |
| | | | 380 ml | |
| 1300 – 1500 | 60 ml/hr x 2 hrs | = | -120 ml | |
| | | | 260 ml | |
| 1500 – 1700 | 80 ml/hr x 2 hrs | = | -160 ml | |
| | | | 100 ml | |
| 1700 – 1800 | 100 ml/hr x 1 hr | = | -100 ml | **At 1800 bag is empty** |
| | | | 0 ml | |

99. You are to dilute 2 g of a powdered medication in a vial to create a concentration of 250 mg/ml. How much diluent should you add?

ml = 1 ml/250 mg x 2000 mg = **8 ml**

100. In the previous question, if the doctor has ordered a 50 mg dose of the medication, how much would you give?

ml = 1 ml/250 mg x 50 mg/d.o. = **0.2 ml**

101. Your 110 lb patient has medication ordered at 60 mg/Kg per day, in four divided doses. The tablets available are 50 mg, 100 mg, 250 mg, and 500 mg. You are to give the fewest number of tablets possible (do NOT cut tablets if possible), and can use more than one tablet size to make up the dose. Which tablet(s) should be given per dose?

mg/day = 60 mg/Kg x 50 Kg = 3000 mg/day
mg/dose = 3000 mg/day x 1 day/4 doses = 750 mg/dose
**Give one 250 mg and one 500 mg tab per dose.**

102. The medication is available 600 mg in a vial. You must add enough diluent to create a strength of 75 mg per ml. How much should you add to the vial?

    ml = 1 ml/75 mg x 600 mg = **8 ml**

103. The doctor has ordered a 250 mg dose every 8 hours for 7 days. The medication comes in 100 mg and 50 mg tablets. How many of each would you need to order for a 7-day supply?

    Doses = 3 doses/day x 7 days = 21 doses
    Each dose one 50 mg & two 100 mg tabs. Therefore, will need:
    2 x 21 = **42   100 mg tablets**
    1 x 21 = **21   50 mg tablets**

104. Penicillin 600,000 units IM is ordered for your patient. PCN is available in a vial containing one million units per ml. How much has the doctor ordered you to give?

    ml = 1 ml/1,000,000 units x 600,000 units/d.o. = **0.6 ml**

105. The medication is available 500 mg in 2 ml. You are to dilute this with 50 ml of NS, then give a 60 mg dose every 6 hours. How much will you give the patient per dose?

    ml = 52 ml/500 mg x 60 mg = **6.2 ml per dose**

106. The doctor has ordered iii grains of a medication which is available 130 mg/ml. How much will you give?

    ml = 1 ml/130 mg x 60 mg/gr x 3 gr/d.o. = **1.4 ml**

107. A powdered medication is available 300 mg in a vial. You must add enough diluent to create a concentration of 50 mg/ml. How much diluent will you add?

    ml = 1 ml/50 mg x 300 mg = **6 ml**

108. How much of the newly reconstituted medication in the previous problem would you draw up to give a 75 mg dose?

ml = 1 ml/50 mg x 75 mg = **1.5 ml**

109. Again based on the medication in problem 107, how much of the medication will be present in 3.5 ml?

mg = 50 mg/1 ml x 3.5 ml = **175 mg**

110. The doctor has ordered 500 mcg of a medication, which is available at your facility only as 0.125 mg tablets. How many tablets will you need to give?

tabs = 1 tab/0.125 mg x 1 mg/1000 mcg x 500 mcg/d.o. = **4 tabs**

111. The patient is to get 1 g per day of a medication, in four divided doses. The medication is available in 125 mg capsules. How many capsules will your patient receive per dose?

caps = 1 cap/125 mg x 1000 mg/1 g x 1 g/day x 1 day/4 doses = **2 caps**

112. The doctor has ordered 12 mg/Kg every 6 hours for your 110 pound patient. Tablets available are 150 mg. How many tablets will your patient receive in one day?

tabs/dose = 1 tab/150 mg x 12 mg/Kg x 50 Kg = 4 tabs/dose
tabs/day = 4 tabs/6 hours x 24 hours/1 day = **16 tabs per day**

113. The medication is available in 15 mg, 30 mg, 60 mg, and 100 mg tablets. It is also available in a solution with a concentration of 50 mg/ml. Your patient, who weighs 35 Kg, has the medication ordered at 4 mg/Kg. Would you give tablets or the solution, and why?

mg = 4 mg/Kg x 35 Kg = 140 mg is patient's ordered dose.
Using tabs, we can come within 5 mg of the order:
One 100 mg + one 30 mg + one 15 mg tab = 145 mg, OR
Two 60 mg + one 15 mg tab = 135 mg

Using the solution: ml = 1 ml/50 mg x 140 mg = 2.8 ml

**We would use the solution, because then we can give the exact dose ordered.**

114. For the previous problem, calculate how much of the available medication you would give.

ml = 1 ml/50 mg x 140 mg = **2.8 ml**

115. The patient has an oral, liquid form of morphine ordered hourly prn (as needed) for pain. The medication is available 20 mg/ml. The doctor's order reads 5 mg for mild pain, 10 mg for moderate pain, and 20 mg for severe pain. During your shift, you dose the patient twice for mild pain, four times for moderate pain, and twice for severe pain. How many ml of the medication did you give on your shift?

| mild pain | mg | = | 5 mg/dose | x | 2 doses | = | 10 mg |
|-----------|-----|---|-----------|---|---------|---|-------|
| moderate pain | | | 10 mg/dose | x | 4 doses | = | 40 mg |
| severe pain | | | 20 mg/dose | x | 2 doses | = | 40 mg |
| | | | | | | TOTAL: | 90 mg |

ml = 1 ml/20 mg x 90 mg = **4.5 ml**

116. An oral solution is available 5 g in 100 ml. The doctor has ordered 250 mg. How much will you give?

ml = 100 ml/5000 mg x 250 mg = **5 ml**

117. The order is for 6 mg of a medication which comes 4 mg/ml in a 10 ml vial. How much will you give your patient?

ml = 1 ml/4 mg x 6 mg/d.o. = **1.5 ml**

118. The ordered potassium comes only in a powdered form with 20 mEq in each small packet, which must be dissolved in 15 ml of fluid. The patient is to get 30 mEq of potassium every 8 hours. How many ml will he get per day?

ml/day = 15 ml/20 mEq x 30 mEq/8 hr x 24 hr/1 day = **67.5 ml/day**

119. You are to add 800 mg of a medication to an IV bag, using a reconstituted solution with a concentration of 500 mg in 8 ml. How much will you add?

ml = 8 ml/500 mg x 800 mg = **12.8 ml**

120. The medication comes as a 100 mg powder. You are to add enough diluent to create a concentration of 25 mg/ml. How much will you add?

ml = 1 ml/25 mg x 100 mg = **4 ml**

121. You are to give 1 g of a medication in four divided doses. How much will you give per dose?

mg/dose = 1000 mg/1 g x 1 g/4 doses = **250 mg/dose**

122. The doctor has ordered 2 g daily in four divided doses. 250 mg tablets are available. How many tablets would you need for a 10-day supply?

tabs = 1 tab/250 mg x 2000 mg/day x 10 days = **80 tabs**, OR
tabs/dose = 1 tab/250 mg x 2000 mg/day x 1 day/4 doses = 2 tabs/dose
tabs/10 days = 2 tabs/dose x 4 doses/day x 10 days = **80 tabs**

123. The ordered medication is available in a concentration of 0.03 mg/ml. The doctor has ordered 90 mcg. How much will you give (in ml)?

ml = 1 ml/0.03 mg x 1 mg/1000 mcg x 90 mcg = **3 ml**

124. The general rule is to give the fewest number of tablets needed to provide the ordered dose, and to avoid cutting tablets if possible. The patient has an order for ¾ gr of medication. The medication is available in 15, 30, and 60 mg scored tablets. How will you give the dose? (Remember, you can use more than one size tablet to create the ordered dose.)

MD ordered mg = 60 mg/1 gr x 0.75 gr = 45 mg
**Give one 15 mg and one 30 mg tab** = 45 mg


125. The patient is to receive continuous feeding through his G tube, starting with a 300 ml bag. He is to start at 30 ml/hr, and you are to increase the rate hourly by 10 ml/hr, checking residual every two hours and stopping the feeding for one hour if there is an hour's worth or more of feeding (at the current rate) in the residual. Maximum rate per the doctor's order is to be 60 ml/hr. If you start the feeding at 1000, at what time will you need to hang a new bag, assuming no excessive residual?

|            |            |   |       |   |          |
|------------|------------|---|-------|---|----------|
|            |            |   |       |   | 300 ml   |
| 1000 – 1100 | 30 ml/hr   | x | 1 hr  | = | - 30 ml  |
|            |            |   |       |   | 270 ml   |
| 1100 – 1200 | 40 ml/hr   | x | 1 hr  | = | - 40 ml  |
|            |            |   |       |   | 230 ml   |
| 1200 – 1300 | 50 ml/hr   | x | 1 hr  | = | -50 ml   |
|            |            |   |       |   | 180 ml   |
| 1300 – 1600 | 60 ml/hr   | x | 3 hr  | = | -180 ml  |
|            |            |   |       |   | 0 ml     |

**At 1600, a new bag will need to be hung.**


126. The doctor has ordered 600,000 units of PCN every 6 hours for the patient. The PCN comes in a vial with a concentration of 2 million units in 5 ml. How much will the patient receive per day?

ml/day = 5 ml/2,000,000 units x 600,000 units/6 hr x 24 hr/day = **6 ml/day**

127.  Order: 1/6 gr
      Available: Elixir with a concentration of 10 mg/2 ml.
      How much has been ordered?

      ml = 2 ml/10 mg x 60 mg/1 gr x 0.16667 gr = **2 ml**


128.  The ordered sliding scale is:

      | | |
      |---|---|
      | 0 – 150 | 0 units of regular insulin |
      | 150 – 249 | 3 units |
      | 250 – 349 | 5 units |
      | 350 – 400 | 8 units |
      | Over 400 | 10 units and call the doctor |

      You check your patient's blood sugar, and it is 323. The insulin comes in a concentration of 50 units per ml. Following the sliding scale, how much will you give your patient?

      ml = 1 ml/50 units x 5 units = **0.1 ml**


129.  The patient is to receive 1.5 g of medication daily, in six divided doses. The medication comes 5 g in a 250 ml bag of IV fluids. How much will the patient receive per dose?

      ml/dose = 250 ml/5000 mg x 1500 mg/day x 1 day/6 doses = **12.5 ml/dose**


130.  The doctor has ordered 750 mg of a medication in a 100 ml IV bag which will be given over a one hour period once daily. You are to reconstitute the medication to create a concentration of 150 mg/ml before adding it to the bag. How much diluent will you use?

      ml = 1 ml/150 mg x 750 mg = **5 ml**


131.  Your patient is to receive a medication at 12 mg/Kg per day, with a dose given every 8 hours. Your patient weighs 99 pounds. How much will she get per dose?

      mg = 12 mg/Kg x 45 Kg = 540 mg/day
      mg = 540 mg/day x 1 day/3 doses = **180 mg/dose**

132. Order: 30 mg
     Available: 500 mcg/ml
     How much will you give?

     ml = 1 ml/500 mcg x 1000 mcg/mg x 30 mg/d.o. = **60 ml**


133. Order: 300 mg
     Available: 10 ml vial with 2 g of medication in it
     How much will you give?

     ml = 10 ml/2000 mg x 300 mg = **1.5 ml**


134. You have reconstituted a powdered medication and how have a 10 ml vial containing 3 g of medication. The doctor wants 750 mg in a 100 ml bag of IV solution. How much of your reconstituted medication should you add to the bag?

     ml = 10 ml/3000 mg x 750 mg/d.o. = **2.5 ml**


135. You have received an order for your patient of 1/120 gr of a medication. How much is that, in mg?

     mg = 60 mg/1 gr x 0.00833 gr = 0.499 mg = **0.5 mg**


136. A powdered medication comes 400 mg in a vial. You are to add enough of a diluent to the vial to create a 125 mg/ml concentration. How much diluent will you add?

     ml = 1 ml/125 mg x 400 mg = **3.2 ml**


137. The doctor has ordered 60 mg of a medication which is available 3 mg/ml. How many tsp will the patient receive?

     ml = 1 ml/3 mg x 60 mg = 20 ml
     tsp = 1 tsp/5 ml x 20 ml = **4 tsp**

138. The patient is to receive 25 mg/Kg per day in four divided doses. How much will the patient receive per dose? (The patient weighs 58 pounds.)

mg = 25 mg/Kg x 1 Kg/2.2 lb x 58 lb = 659 mg/day
mg/dose = 659 mg/day x 1 day/4 doses = **164.75 = 164.8 mg/dose**


139. The order is for 1.5 g of medication to be given daily, divided into one dose every four hours. How much should be given per dose?

mg/dose = 1500 mg/day x 1 day/6 doses = **250 mg/dose**


140. You are to give a tube feeding at 0900, starting at 20 ml/hr and increasing the rate every 2 hours by 10 ml/hr. At what time will you reach the ordered rate of 70 ml/hr?

| | |
|---|---|
| 0900 – 1100 | 20 ml/hr |
| 1100 – 1300 | 30 ml/hr |
| 1300 – 1500 | 40 ml/hr |
| 1500 – 1700 | 50 ml/hr |
| 1700 – 1900 | 60 ml/hr |

**Changes to 70 ml/hr at 1900.**

141. Order: 1/6 gr
Available: medication containing 1/120 gr per ml
How many ml has the doctor ordered?

ml = 1 ml/0.00833 gr x 0.16667 gr/d.o. = **20 ml**


142. Your patient is to get Roxanol, a liquid form of morphine, prn for pain. The order reads: 5 mg for mile pain (1-3 on 1-10 pain scale), 10 mg for mild pain (4-7 on the scale), and 20 mg for severe pain (8-10 on the scale), hourly as needed. During your shift, you give 4 doses for mild pain, 2 for moderate pain, and 4 for severe pain. The medication is available 20 mg/ml. How much did you give, in ml, during your shift?

5 mg x 4 = 20 mg          20 + 20 + 80 = 120 mg
10 mg x 2 = 20 mg
20 mg x 4 = 80 mg

ml = 1 ml/20 mg x 120 mg = **6 ml**

143. Order: 300 mg of a medication
     Available: elixir 40 mg/ml
     How much will you give?

     ml = 1 ml/40 mg x 300 mg = **7.5 ml**

144. The doctor has ordered 3 grains of phenobarbital for a patient's agitation. The medication is available in a liquid form of 65 mg/ml. How much will you give?

     mg = 60 mg/gr x 3 gr = 180 mg
     ml = 1 ml/65 mg x 180 mg = 2.769 = **2.8 ml**

145. Your 206.8 pound patient is to receive a medication ordered at 12 mg/Kg/24 hours, in three divided doses. The medication comes as 375 mg tablets. How many tablets will he get per dose?

     mg = 12 mg/Kg x 94 Kg = 1128 mg/3 doses = 376 mg/dose
     So he will get **1 tablet per dose**.

146. The medication comes as 0.5 g powder in a 10 ml vial. You are to create a concentration of 250 mg/ml. How much diluent must you add?

     ml = 1 ml/250 mg x 500 mg = **2 ml**

147. Order: 750 mg of a medication
     Available: 1 g in a 5 ml vial
     How much will you give?

     ml = 5 ml/1000 mg x 750 mg = 3750/1000 = 3.75 = **3.8 ml**

148. The patient is to receive a tube feeding of 630 ml of Jevity. Because she has not previously had tube feedings, the doctor is not sure what rate she will tolerate. He therefore orders the feeding to begin at 20 ml/hr, increasing 10 ml/hr every hour, to a maximum rate of 80 ml/hr. You start the feeding at 0800. At what time will the bag be empty?

| | | |
|---|---|---|
| | | 630 ml |
| 0800-0900 | 20 ml/hr | - 20 ml |
| | | 610 ml |
| 0900-1000 | 30 ml/hr | -30 ml |
| | | 580 ml |
| 1000-1100 | 40 ml/hr | -40 ml |
| | | 540 ml |
| 1100-1200 | 50 ml/hr | -50 ml |
| | | 490 ml |
| 1200-1300 | 60 ml/hr | -60 ml |
| | | 430 ml |
| 1300-1400 | 70 ml/hr | -70 ml |
| | | 360 ml |
| 1400-1800 | 80 ml/hr | -320 ml |
| | | 40 ml |
| 1800-1830 | 80 ml/hr | -40 ml |
| | | 0 |

The bag will be empty at **1830**.

149. The doctor has ordered 500 mg of a medication four times daily. The medication arrives from the pharmacy in the form of 250 mg tablets. How many tablets will be needed for a three-day supply?

tabs = 1 tab/250 mg x 500 mg/dose x 4 doses/day x 3 days = **24 tabs**

150. The order is for 1 unit/Kg of insulin for your 200-pound patient. How many units will the patient receive? (Remember, for insulin, answer must be in whole numbers.)

units = 1 unit/Kg x 1 Kg/2.2 lb. x 200 lb = **91 units**

# IV DOSAGE CALCULATIONS

1.  Your patient is to receive 3 liters of maintenance fluids in the next 12 hours. At what rate should you set the pump?

    ml/hr = 1000 ml/liter x 3 liters/12 hours = **250 ml/hr**

2.  Using 15 gtt/ml tubing, what would the drip rate be for problem 1?

    gtt/min = 15 gtt/ml x 250 ml/60 min = **63 gtt/min**

3.  What tubing (macro or micro) would you use for each of the following?

    a.  A frail 72-year-old female with fluids ordered at 75 ml/hr **micro**
    b.  A 27-year-old male with pneumonia who is to get antibiotics at 100 ml/hr **macro**
    c.  A 10-year-old child with normal saline ordered at 60 ml/hr **micro**
    d.  A 42-year-old post-surgical patient receiving a blood transfusion **macro**

4.  Your patient is to receive the full dose of 250 ml of an antibiotic within the two-hour window prior to his scheduled surgery. Surgery is scheduled for noon. You therefore hang the antibiotic at 1000 at 125 ml an hour. At 1045, the patient has to be disconnected from his IV for an MRI. He does not return until 1115. At what rate do you have to set the pump now to ensure all of the antibiotic will be infused prior to the patient's scheduled surgery time?

    ml = 125 ml/hr x 1 hr/60 min x 45 min = 93.75 ml has infused when IV is disconnected. When pt returns, he has 156.25 ml left to infuse, and only 45 minutes until his scheduled surgery, so pump must be set at ml/hr = 156.25 ml/45 min x 60 min/hr = **208.3 ml/hr.**

5.  Mr. Lawler has 900 ml of NS to infuse at 85 ml/hr. How long will it take to infuse?

    hr = 1 hr/85 ml x 900 ml = 10.588 hours
    min = 60 min/1 hr x 0.59 hr = 35.4 min = 35 min
    So it will take **10 hours 35 minutes** to infuse.

6.  What hourly dosage of heparin will your patient receive if he is getting the usual 100:1 (25,000 units/250 ml) heparin at 14.7 ml/hr?

    units/hr = 25,000 units/250 ml x 14.7 ml/hr = **1470 units/hr**

7.  Calculate the flow rate and drip rate for a patient receiving 400 ml in two and a half hours. Tubing available is 20 gtt/ml.

    ml/hr = 400 ml/2.5 hr = **160 ml/hr**
    gtt/min = 20 gtt/ml x 160 ml/60 min = **53 gtt/min**

8.  The patient has 500 ml to be infused in 6 hours. Calculate the drip rate, using 15 gtt/ml tubing.

    500 ml/6 hr = 83.3 ml/hr is the flow rate
    gtt/min = 15 gtt/ml x 83.3 ml/60 min = **21 gtt/min**

9.  Ms. Snowden is to get 4 mg of a medication per Kg of body weight. She weighs 159 pounds. The medication is then to be diluted in 150 ml NS and infused at 26 mg/hr. What is the hourly rate?

    mg = 4 mg/Kg x 1 Kg/2.2 lb x 159 lb = 289.1 mg ordered
    ml/hr = 150 ml/289.1 mg x 26 mg/hr = **13.5 ml/hr**

10. Mr. Peterson is very ill. He has D5W infusing at 100 ml/hr. The doctor has also ordered levofloxacin 1 g in 250 ml D5W twice daily, to infuse over 90 minutes, Ancef 1.5 g in 150 ml every eight hours, to infuse over an hour, and Aztreonam 1 g in 100 ml every six hours, to infuse over 30 minutes. Calculate the flow rate for each of the antibiotics, and determine Mr. Peterson's 24-hour parenteral intake.

D5W 100 ml/hr x 16 hr = 1600 ml
Lev 250 ml/dose x 2 doses = 500 ml (given over 3 hours total)
Anc 150 ml/dose x 3 doses = 450 ml (given over three hours total)
Aztr 100 ml/dose x 4 doses = 400 ml (given over 2 hours total)

1600 + 500 + 450 + 400 = **2950 ml**
Levaquin 250 ml/1.5 hr = **166.7 ml/hr**
Ancef **150 ml/hr** (given in the problem)
Aztreonam 100 ml/30 min x 60 min/hr = **200 ml/hr**

11. What is the needed hourly rate if 100 ml is to be infused in 35 minutes?

ml/hr = 100 ml/35 min x 60 min/hr = **171.4 ml/hr**

12. Your patient is receiving a magnesium rider at 25 ml/hr. The concentration of the rider is 5 g in 100 ml. What is his hourly dosage?

mg/hr = 5000 mg/100 ml x 25 ml/hr = **1250 mg/hr**

13. Mr. Aaronson is to receive 2 L of D5 1/2 NS over the next 12 hours. What will the hourly rate be?

ml/hr = 2000 ml/12 hr = **166.7 ml/hr**

14. Mr. Franklin is receiving his IV medication at 200 mg/hr. He is receiving 2 g of the medication in 250 ml of NS. Another medication is to be hung as soon as the current medication is completely infused. It is now 1400. At what time should you be able to hang the new medication?

hr = 1 hr/200 mg x 2000 mg = 10 hours

**Can hang the new medication at 2400.**

15. Determine the flow rate needed to infuse the medication in the previous problem in half the time you calculated for the problem.

ml/hr = 250 ml/5 hr = **50 ml/hr**

16. The medication is infusing at 75 ml/hr. Calculate the drip rate separately using 10, 15, 20, and 60 gtt/ml tubing.

gtt/min = 10 gtt/ml x 75 ml/60 min = 12.5 = **13 gtt/min**
gtt/min = 15 gtt/ml x 75 ml/60 min = 18.75 = **19 gtt/min**
gtt/min = 20 gtt/ml x 75 ml/60 min = **25 gtt/min**
gtt/min = 60 gtt/ml x 75 ml/60 min = **75 gtt/min**

**Questions 17 – 19 are based on the following scenario:**

**Your patient is to receive one liter of IV fluids over 12 hours. You hang the bag at 0200. When you check the bag at 0530, you realize only 380 ml have infused.**

17. What flow rate should have been set per the original order?

ml/hr = 1000 ml/12 hr = **83.3 ml/hr**

18. At what flow rate was it actually infusing?

ml/hr = 380 ml/3.5 hr = **108.6 ml/hr**

19. At what rate should you now set the pump to be sure the one liter finishes infusing at 1400?

    ml/hr = 620 ml/8.5 hr = **72.9 ml/hr**

20. Mr. Anodin is to receive 700 ml of fluid at 45 ml/hr. How long will it require to infuse?

    hr = 1 hr/45 ml x 700 ml = 15.56 hr
    min = 60 min/hr x 0.56 hr = 33.6 min
    It will take **15 hr 34 min** to infuse.

21. Calculate the flow rate and drip rate for a 100 ml dose of a medication which is to infuse in 25 minutes.

    ml/hr = 100 ml/25 min x 60 min/1 hr = **240 ml/hr**
    gtt/min = 10 gtt/ml x 240 ml/60 min = **40 gtt/min**

22. Mr. Baker has orders for maintenance fluids to infuse one liter every 9 hours. You hang a fresh one-liter bag at 0700. At 0900, Mr. Baker leaves the floor for a test. You assume his IV has gone with him and do not realize until two hours and 15 minutes after he returns at 0945 that he was disconnected from his IV fluids and never reconnected. At what rate must you now set the pump to meet the 9-hour infusion deadline for this bag of fluid?

    Was initially at 1000 ml/9 hr = 111.1 ml/hr, so at 0900, 222.2 ml are in.

    Bag should have run from 0700 – 1600. You have lost the time from 0900 to 1200 (back to the floor at 0945 + 2 hr 15 min = 1200). You have four hours left to infuse the rest of the liter bag, from 1200 to 1600. You have 1000 ml - 222.2 ml = 777.8 ml left, so

    ml/hr = 777.8 ml/4 hr = **194.5 ml/hr**

23. The doctor has ordered a medication which comes in a vial with a concentration of 350 mg/ml. You are to add 2.1 g of this medication to a 100 ml bag of NS and infuse it in 30 minutes. At what rate will you set the pump?

    ml = 1 ml/350 mg x 2100 mg = 6 ml
    ml/hr = 106 ml/30 min x 60 min/hr = **212 ml/hr**

24. 750 ml of fluid is infusing at 33 gtt/min using 15 gtt/ml tubing. What is its flow rate?

    ml/hr = 1 ml/15 gtt x 33 gtt/min x 60 min/hr = **132 ml/hr**

25. Heparin 10,000 units in 100 ml is infusing at 12.9 ml/hr. What is the hourly dosage?

    units/hr = 10,000 units/100 ml x 12.9 ml/hr = **1290 units/hr**

26. You are to reconstitute 1 g of a powdered medication with 20 ml of sterile water. How much of this reconstituted medication will you add to a 100 ml bag of D5W to create the doctor's order of 250 mg of the medication?

    ml = 20 ml/1 g x 1 g/1000 mg x 250 mg = **5 ml**

27. In the previous problem, what flow rate would you set to give 40 mg/hour?

    ml/hr = 105 ml/250 mg x 40 mg/hr = **16.8 ml/hr**

28. Mrs. Jackson is receiving D5 1/2 NS at 150 ml/hr, antibiotic A 500 mg in 50 ml every six hours (infuse over 30 minutes), antibiotic B 2 g in 150 ml three times daily (infuse over one hour), and a potassium rider of 200 ml (infuse over 90 minutes). She is on strict I&O. What is her 24-hour parenteral intake?

    | | | | | | |
    |---|---|---|---|---|---|
    | D5 1/2 NS | 150 ml/hr | x | 17.5 hr | = | 2625 ml |
    | Abx. A | 50 ml/dose | x | 4 doses | = | 200 ml (over 2 hr total) |
    | Abx. B | 150 ml/dose | x | 3 doses | = | 450 ml (over 3 hr total) |
    | Potassium | 200 ml (over 1.5 hr) | | | | |

    2625 + 200 + 450 + 200 = **3475 ml**

29. With 10 gtt/ml tubing, determine flow rate and drip rate for each of the fluids in the previous problem.

D5 1/2 NS FR **150 ml/hr** (given in problem); DR 10 gtt/ml x 150 ml/hr = **25 gtt/min**
Abx. A FR 50 ml/30 min x 60 min/hr = **100 ml/hr**;
DR 10 gtt/ml x 100 ml/60 min = **17 gtt/min**
Abx. B FR **150 ml/hr** (given in problem); DR same as for D5 1/2 NS = **25 gtt/min**
Potassium FR 200 ml/1.5 hr = **133.3 ml/hr**; DR 10 gtt/ml x 133.3 ml/60 min = **22 gtt/min**

30. The patient is to receive a 75 ml dose of medication IV at 128.6 ml/hr. How many minutes will it take to infuse?

min. = 60 min/1 hr x 1 hr/128.6 ml x 75 ml = **35 min.**

31. It is now 0835. Your patient has 700 ml of fluid left in a bag running at 55 ml/hr. At what time will the bag be empty?

hr = 1 hr/55 ml x 700 ml = 12.73 hr
min = 60 min/1 hr x 0.73 hr = 44 min
So the bag will take 12 hr 44 min to run in. 0835 + 1244 = 2079
So **the bag will be empty at 2119.**

32. After reconstituting a medication, you have a 10 ml vial containing 500 mg of medication per 2 ml. The doctor has ordered 750 mg of medication be given. How much of the reconstituted medication will you need to use?

ml = 2 ml/500 mg x 750 mg = **3 ml**

33. In the previous problem, you add the needed amount of reconstituted medication to a 50 ml bag. What flow rate will you set to infuse it in 30 minutes?

ml/hr = 53 ml/30 min x 60 min/1 hr = **106 ml/hr**

34. The patient is to receive 100 ml of fluid in 40 minutes. Calculate the flow rate and drip rate.

ml/hr = 100 ml/40 min x 60 min/1 hr = **150 ml/hr**
gtt/min = 10 gtt/ml x 150 ml/60 min = **25 gtt/min**

35. The patient has 500 ml of fluid to be infused, using 15 gtt/ml tubing and running at 40 gtt/min. How long will it take to infuse?

min = 1 min/40 gtt x 15 gtt/ml x 500 ml = 187.5 min = **3 hr 8 min**

36. Heparin is infusing at 9.8 ml/hr. The solution infusing has 10,000 units heparin in 100 ml D5W. What is the hourly dosage?

units/hr = 10,000 units/100 ml x 9.8 ml/hr = **980 units/hr**

**Questions 37 and 38 are based on the following:**

**The antibiotic is to be reconstituted to create a concentration of 500 mg in 100 ml. The available antibiotic comes in a 5 ml vial containing 2 g.**

37. How much of the available antibiotic must be added to the 100 ml bag to create the desired concentration? (Take your answer to hundredths.)

ml = 5 ml/2000 mg x 500 mg = **1.25 ml**

38. At what rate would you set the pump for the newly reconstituted medication to infuse in 45 minutes?

ml/hr = 101.25 ml/45 min x 60 min/1 hr = **135 ml/hr**

39. It is 0800. There are 720 ml remaining in the bag of ½ NS, which is infusing at 70 ml/hr. At what time will you need to hang a new bag, assuming you let the old bag run until empty?

    hr = 1 hr/70 ml x 720 ml = 10.29 hr = 10 hr 17 min

    So **will need to hang a new bag at 1817.**


40. If a patient has 50 ml to infuse in 25 minutes, at what rate should you set the pump?

    ml/hr = 50 ml/25 min x 60 min/1 hr = **120 ml/hr**


41. A liter of D5.2NS is to infuse at 42 gtt/min, using tubing labeled 20 gtt/ml. How long will it take to infuse?

    min = 1 min/42 gtt x 20 gtt/1 ml x 1000 ml = 476 min = **7 hr 56 min**


42. 250 ml of a medication are to be infused in one hour. The set is calibrated at 15 gtt/ml. What is the drip rate?

    gtt/min = 15 gtt/ml x 250 ml/60 min = **63 gtt/min**


**Questions 43 and 44 are based on the following information:**

**Available medication is 1.5 g in a 10 ml vial. The doctor has ordered a 600 mg dose.**

43. How much should you add to the 100 ml bag of D5W to create the ordered dose?

    ml = 10 ml/1.5 g x 1 g/1000 mg x 600 mg = **4 ml**


44. What flow rate would you set if the medication is to infuse in 30 minutes?

    ml/hr = 104 ml/30 min x 60 min/hr = **208 ml/hr**

45. A liter of D5.45NS is to infuse in 9 hours. Calculate the flow rate and drip rate. Only microdrip tubing is available.

   ml/hr = 1000 ml/9 hr = **111.1 ml/hr**
   gtt/min = 60 gtt/ml x 111.11 ml/60 min = **111 gtt/min**

46. The doctor has ordered a 500 ml bolus of NS. It will infuse at 60 gtt/min, using 20 gtt/ml tubing. How long will it take to infuse?

   min = 1 min/60 gtt x 20 gtt/ml x 500 ml = 166.67 min = 167 min = **2 hr 47 min**

47. In the previous problem, what is the flow rate?

   ml/hr = 1 ml/20 gtt x 60 gtt/min x 60 min/1 hr = **180 ml/hr**, OR
   ml/hr = 500 ml/166.7 min x 60 min/1 hr = **180 ml/hr**

48. The patient is on strict I&O. In the past 24 hours, he has had emesis of 380 ml and diarrhea of 650 ml. You are now to calculate his parenteral intake over the same period of time. He is receiving D5W at 125 ml/hr, antibiotic A 2 g in 150 ml every eight hours (infused over 60 minutes) and antibiotic B 500 mg in 50 ml every six hours (infused over 30 minutes). What is his 24- hour parenteral intake?

   D5W 125 ml/hr x 19 hr = 2375 ml
   Abx. A 150 ml/dose x 3 doses = 450 ml (over 3 hrs total)
   Abx. B 50 ml/dose x 4 doses = 200 ml (over 2 hrs total)
   2375 + 450 + 200 = **3025 ml**

49. A patient is to receive a 500 ml bolus of fluid over a 3-hour period just prior to surgery scheduled at 1100. You hang the bag at 0745. At 0930 the IV is discontinued as the patient is taken from the floor for an Xray, returning at 1015. At what rate should you restart the IV fluids to ensure complete infusion by 1100?

   Initially hung at 166.7 ml/hr (500 ml/3 hr). At 0930, 291.7 ml have run in, leaving 208.3 ml. At 1015, with only 45 min left, must set pump at:

   ml/hr = 208.3 ml/45 min x 60 min/1 hr = **277.7 ml/hr**

50. 1000 ml of LR is infusing at 60 gtt/min using tubing labeled 20 gtt/ml. How long will it take for complete infusion?

min = 1 min/60 gtt x 20 gtt/ml x 1000 ml = 333 min = **5 hr 33 min**

51. Calculate the flow rate and drip rate necessary to infuse 500 ml of IV fluids in two and one half hours. Tubing is calibrated at 10 gtt/ml.

ml/hr = 500 ml/2.5 hr = **200 ml/hr**
gtt/min = 10 gtt/ml x 200 ml/60 min = **33 gtt/min**

52. The antibiotic comes as 2 g powder in a 10 ml vial. You are to reconstitute it using 8 ml of sterile water, then add it to a 50 ml bag of D5W to meet the doctor's order. The order is for 500 mg of the antibiotic every 8 hours. How much of the reconstituted fluid will you add to the bag?

ml = 8 ml/2 g x 1 g/1000 mg x 500 mg = **2 ml**

53. Your patient is receiving D5 1/2 NS at 180 ml/hr. The doctor has also ordered two antibiotics: antibiotic A 500 mg in 50 ml every 6 hours (infuse over 30 min.), and antibiotic B 1.5 g in 100 ml every 8 hours (infuse over 60 min.). How much IV fluid will infuse in 24 hours?

| D5 1/2 NS | A | B | |
|---|---|---|---|
| 180 ml/hr | 50 ml/dose | 100 ml/dose | |
| x 19 hr | x 4 doses | x 3 doses | |
| 3420 ml + | 200 ml + | 300 ml | =**3920 ml** |
| | - 2 hr | - 3 hr | |

54. For the three IV fluids in the previous problem, what are the flow rate and drip rate of each? Tubing size: 15 gtt/ml.

D5 1/2 NS **180 ml/hr** (given in problem); gtt/min = 15 gtt/ml x 180 ml/60 min = **45 gtt/min**
A      ml/hr = 50 ml/30 min x 60 min/hr = **100 ml/hr**; gtt/min =
      15 gtt/ml x 100 ml/60 min = **25 gtt/min**
B      ml/hr = **100 ml/hr** (given in problem); gtt/min =
      15 gtt/ml x 100 ml/60 min = **25 gtt/min**

55. Your patient is to receive 2 liters of fluid overnight, all to be infused prior to surgery scheduled for 0900 tomorrow morning. You hang the first liter bag at 2000 and the infusion is complete at 0200. You hang the second liter bag immediately (at 0200). At 0515 the pump alarms, and you note the site has infiltrated at some point with only 450 ml infused. By the time you start a new IV site and restart the infusion, it is 0545.

    a.    At what rate did the first liter bag infuse?

        ml/hr = 1000 ml/6 hours = **166.7 ml/hr**

    b.    At what rate will you need to set the pump at 0545 to be sure the second liter is infused prior to surgery?

        1000 ml – 450 ml infused = 550 ml left to infuse in 3.25 hours
        ml/hr = 550 ml/3.25 hours = **169.2 ml/hr**

56. You hang a 500 ml bolus at 0700, to infuse at 135 ml/hr. At what time will the bag be empty?

    hr = 1 hr/135 ml = 3.7 hours = 3 hours 42 min
    so bag will be empty at **1042**

57. The liter bag of Lactated Ringer's is infusing at 22 gtt/min using 20 gtt/ml tubing. How long will it take to infuse?

    min = 1 min/22 gtt x 20 gtt/ml x 1000 ml = 909 min = **15 hr 9 min**

58. The medication comes in a 10 ml vial with a concentration of 120 mg/ml. The doctor's order is for 1 g in 100 ml to be given over 90 min.

    a.    How much of the medication will need to be added to the 100 ml bag to follow the order?
        ml = 1 ml/120 mg x 1000 mg = **8.3 ml**

    b.    At what rate will you infuse the medication?
        ml/hr = 108.3 ml/90 min x 60 min/1 hr = **72.2 ml/hr**

59. Calculate the flow rate for the following:

    a.  50 ml in 15 minutes
        ml/hr = 50 ml/15 min x 60 min/1 hr = **200 ml/hr**

    b.  100 ml in 45 minutes
        ml/hr = 100 ml/45 min x 60 min/1 hr = **133.3 ml/hr**

    c.  250 ml in 90 minutes
        ml/hr = 250 ml/90 min x 60 min/1 hr = **166.7 ml/hr**

60. The pharmacy sent up three antibiotics, all scheduled to be hung at 0900. The protocol at your facility states all fluids must be administered within 45 minutes of their scheduled time. The fluids ordered are A, to infuse over 90 minutes; B, to infuse over 60 minutes; and C, to infuse over 30 minutes. At what time would you hang each to follow facility policy?

    **0815-0845 C; 0845 – 0945 B; 0945 A (possibility #1) OR 0815-0915 B; 0915-0945 C; 0945 A (poss.#2)**

61. The ordered medication is available in a 10 ml vial containing 500 mg/ml. The doctor has ordered 3.5 g in 250 ml ½ NS to be infused over 90 minutes, using 10 gtt/ml tubing.

    a.  How much medication will you add to the NS?
        ml = 1 ml/500 mg x 3500 mg = **7 ml**

    b.  At what rate will you set the pump?
        ml/hr = 257 ml/1.5 hr = **171.3 ml/hr**

    c.  What would the drip rate be?
        gtt/min = 10 gtt/ml x 171.3 ml/60 min = **29 gtt/min**

62. The liter bag of D5 1/2 NS is infusing at 85 ml/hr. The nurse on the previous shift states she just hung it at 0530. At what time should you be prepared to hang a new bag?

    hr = 1 hr/85 ml x 1000 ml = 11.76 hr = 11hr 46 min, so at **1716**

63. The patient is receiving NS at 150 ml an hour. He has a 50 ml potassium rider ordered (to infuse over 90 minutes), and two antibiotics. Antibiotic A 500 mg in 100 ml is ordered every 8 hours (to infuse over 30 minutes), and antibiotic B 1 g in 200 ml is ordered every 12 hours (to infuse over 90 minutes). Total 24-hour parenteral intake?

| NS | | K⁺ | | A | | B | |
|---|---|---|---|---|---|---|---|
| 150 ml/hr | | 50 ml | | 100 ml | | 200 ml | |
| x 18 hr | | x 1 | | x 3 | | x 2 | |
| 2700 ml | + | 50 ml | + | 300 ml | + | 400 ml | = **3450 ml** |
| | | - 1.5 hr | | -1.5 hr | | - 3 hr | |

64. Calculate the drip rate for the following:

   a. 1000 ml infusing in 12 hours
   gtt/min = 60 gtt/ml x 83.3 ml/60 min = **83 gtt/min**

   b. 750 ml infusing in 6 hours
   gtt/min = 10 gtt/ml x 125 ml/60 min = **21 gtt/min**

   c. 150 ml infusing in 90 minutes
   gtt/min = 10 gtt/ml x 150 ml/90 min = **17 gtt/min**

65. The doctor has ordered 1500 ml of fluid infused within 10 hours. You hang the fluid at 1000. At 1230 the patient's IV is disconnected and he leaves the floor for testing, not returning until 1430. You reconnect his IV immediately. At what rate should you set the pump now, to comply with the order?

   Initial rate was 150 ml/hr, so at 1230, 375 ml has infused, leaving 1125 ml. Ordered ending time: 2000. When pt returns, only 5.5 hours left.

   ml/hr = 1125 ml/5.5 hr = **204.5 ml/hr**

66. The patient has a heparin drip 25,000 units in 250 ml, infusing at 1320 units per hour. What is the flow rate?

   ml/hr = 250 ml/25,000 units x 1320 units/hr = **13.2 ml/hr**

67. A liter bag of D5W is infusing at 34 gtt/min using 15 gtt/ml tubing. What is the flow rate?

    ml/hr = 1 ml/15 gtt x 34 gtt/min x 60 min/hr = **136 ml/hr**

68. In the previous problem, how long will it take to infuse?

    min = 1 min/34 gtt x 15 gtt/ml x 1000 ml = 441 min = **7 hr 21 min**
    **OR** hr = 1 hr/136 ml x 1000 ml = 7.35 hours = 7 hr 21 min

69. Calculate flow rate and drip rate for 250 ml to infuse in 45 minutes.

    ml/hr = 250 ml/45 min x 60 min/hr = **333.3 ml/hr**
    gtt/min = 10 gtt/ml x 333.3 ml/60 min = **56 gtt/min**

70. Your patient has a loading dose of a medication 1500 mg in 250 ml, to infuse in 90 minutes. What is the hourly dosage of this medication?

    mg/hr = 1500 mg/90 min x 60 min/1 hr = **1000 mg/hr**

71. The medication is available 3 g in a 10 ml vial. The doctor has ordered 750 mg be added to a 50 ml bag of D5W and infused every 6 hours (infuse over 30 minutes). How much of the medication should you add to the D5W?

    ml = 10 ml/3000 mg x 750 mg = **2.5 ml**

72. Calculate the flow rate and drip rate for the previous problem.

    ml/hr = 52.5 ml/30 min x 60 min/1 hr = **105 ml/hr**
    gtt/min = 10 gtt/ml x 105 ml/60 min = **18 gtt/min**

73. At 1100, you hang a liter bolus of NS at 110 ml/hr. At what time will the bolus be complete?

    hr = 1 hr/110 ml x 1000 ml = 9.09 hr = 9 hr 5 min, so at **2005** will be done

74. The doctor has ordered NS at a KVO (keep vein open) rate of 20 ml/hr. No IV bag may hang for more than 24 hours, per hospital policy. Available bags: 50 ml, 100 ml, 250 ml, 500 ml, and 1 liter. Which would you choose to hang at 0800, so another does not have to be hung for 24 hours? (Assume no other IV fluids, and unbroken flow.)

    20 ml/hr x 24 hr = 480 ml, so **hang the 500 ml bag**

75. The medication is available in a vial 2 g in 2 ml of fluid. You dilute this with 20 ml of sterile water, then add 1.2 g of it to a 100 ml bag of NS. How much fluid will you add to the bag?

    ml = 22 ml/2000 mg x 1200 mg = **13.2 ml**

76. Order: 500 ml to infuse in 6 hours. Only tubing available is 20 gtt/ml. What are the flow rate and drip rate?

    ml/hr = 500 ml/6 hr = **83.3 ml/hr**
    gtt/min = 20 gtt/ml x 83.3 ml/60 min = **28 gtt/min**

77. A liter bag of NS is infusing at 41 gtt/min, using 20 gtt/ml tubing. How long will it take to infuse?

    min = 1 min/41 gtt x 20 gtt/ml x 1000 ml = 487.8 = 488 min = **8 hr 8 min**

78. In the previous problem, at what rate is the pump set?

    ml/hr = 1 ml/20 gtt x 41 gtt/min x 60 min/1 hr = **123 ml/hr**

79.   The heparin is available 25,000 units in 250 ml. The doctor has ordered the heparin to be infused at 14.3 ml/hr. What is the patient's hourly dosage?

units/hr = 25,000 units/250 ml x 14.3 ml/hr = **1430 units/hr**

80.   The patient is to get a 750 ml bolus of D5 1/2 NS at 60 ml/hr. If you hang it at 0930, at what time will the ordered amount have infused?

hr = 1 hr/60 ml x 750 ml = 12.5 hr, so at **2200** will be complete.

81.   Using 20 gtt/ml tubing and running at 42 gtt/min, how long will it take for a one liter bag of IV fluids to infuse?

min = 1 min/42 gtt x 20 gtt/ml x 1000 ml = 476 min = **7 hr 56 min**

82.   Calculate the flow rate and drip rate of 750 ml infusing in 8 hours. Tubing available: 10 gtt/ml.

ml/hr = 750 ml/8 hr = **93.8 ml/hr**
gtt/min = 10 gtt/ml x 93.8 ml/60 min = 15.6 = **16 gtt/min**

83.   The IV antibiotic ordered contains 1000 mg in 150 ml, infusing in 45 minutes. What is the hourly dosage?

mg/hr = 1000 mg/45 min x 60 min/1 hr = **1333.3 mg/hr**

84.   Patient's meds: D5W at 100 ml/hr, antibiotic A 1000 mg in 100 ml twice daily (infuse over 30 minutes), antibiotic B 2.5 g in 150 ml every 8 hours (infuse over 90 minutes). What is his 24-hour parenteral intake?

| D5W | | A | | B | |
|---|---|---|---|---|---|
| 100 ml/hr | | 100 ml | | 150 ml | |
| X 18.5 hr | | x 2 | | x 3 | |
| 1850 ml | + | 200 ml | + | 450 ml | = **2500 ml** |
| | | - 1 hr | | - 4.5 hr | |

85. Order: 1 liter LR to be hung at 0900 and infused by the scheduled time of surgery at 1500. At 1200 the patient goes down for an MRI and his IV is disconnected for one hour.

    a. What was the initial flow rate when you hung the LR?

    ml/hr = 1000 ml/6 hr = **166.7 ml/hr**

    b. What will the adjusted flow rate be at 1300, in order for the infusion to be complete by 1500?

    At noon, 500 ml is in. At 1300, two hours of time is left, so
    ml/hr = 500 ml/2 hr = **250 ml/hr**

86. Your patient has IV fluids infusing at a KVO rate of 25 ml/hr. Using 15 gtt/ml tubing, calculate the drip rate.

    gtt/min = 15 gtt/ml x 25 ml/60 min = **6 gtt/min**

87. 250 ml of an antibiotic has been ordered, to infuse in 90 minutes. Flow rate and drip rate?

    ml/hr = 250 ml/1.5 hours = **166.7 ml/hr**
    gtt/min = 10 gtt/ml x 166.7 ml/60 min = **28 gtt/min**

88. IV fluids are infusing at 135 ml/hr. Assuming you hung the liter bag of fluids at 0900, at what time will the bag be empty?

    hr = 1 hr/135 ml x 1000 ml = 7.41 hr = 7 hr 25 min
    so the bag will be empty at **1625**

89. The patient has D5 1/2 NS infusing at 125 ml/hr. A 50 ml potassium rider is to be given over 1 hour. The patient also has 100 ml of antibiotic A every 6 hours (infuse over 30 minutes) and 200 ml of antibiotic B twice daily (infuse over 60 minutes). What is his 24-hour parenteral intake?

| D5 1/2 NS | K+ | A | B | |
|---|---|---|---|---|
| 125 ml/hr | 50 ml | 100 ml | 200 ml | |
| X 19 hr | x 1 | x 4 | x 2 | |
| 2375 ml  + | 50 ml  + | 400 ml  + | 400 ml | = **3225 ml** |
| | - 1 hr | - 2 hr | - 2 hr | |

90. What is the drip rate of each IV fluid in the previous problem, using 20 gtt/ml tubing?

D5 1/2 NS 20 gtt/ml x 125 ml/hr = **42 gtt/min**
K+ 20 gtt/ml x 50 ml/60 min = **17 gtt/min**
A 20 gtt/ml x 100 ml/30 min = **67 gtt/min**
B 20 gtt/ml x 200 ml/60 min = **67 gtt/min**

91. The doctor has ordered 750 mg of a medication be added to a 50 ml bag of NS and infused over 30 minutes. The medication must be reconstituted. It is available 3 g in a 10 ml vial.

   a. How much of the medication will you add to the 50 ml bag to follow the doctor's order?
   ml = 10 ml/3000 mg x 750 mg = **2.5 ml**

   b. At what rate will you set the pump to infuse the medication?
   ml/hr = 52.5 ml/30 min x 60 min/1 hr = **105 ml/hr**

92. Heparin is available 10,000 units in 100 ml of D5W. It is infusing into your patient at 13.6 ml/hr. What is the hourly dosage?

units/hr = 10,000 units/100 ml x 13.6 ml/hr = **1360 units/hr**

93. A liter of IV fluids is flowing at 26 gtt/min using 15 gtt/ml tubing.

   a. If you hang the bag at 1130, at what time will you need to hang a new bag? (Assume the old bag is completely empty before a new one is hung.)
   min = 1 min/26 gtt x 15 gtt/ml x 1000 ml = 576.92 = 577 min = 9 hr 37 min
   so will hang new bag at **2107**

   b. At what flow rate is it infusing?
   ml/hr = 1 ml/15 gtt x 26 gtt/min x 60 min/1 hr = **104 ml/hr**

94. You are to add NS to a vial to create a concentration of 500 mg/ml. The 10 ml vial contains 4 g of a powdered medication. How much fluid do you need to add?

   ml = 1 ml/500 mg x 4000 mg = **8 ml**

95. A liter bag of fluid is infusing at 90 ml/hr. The only tubing available is 10 gtt/ml. What is the drip rate for this fluid?

   gtt/min = 10 gtt/ml x 90 ml/60 min = **15 gtt/min**

96. 750 mg of a medication in 100 ml NS is to infuse at 60 mg/hr. What is the flow rate?

   ml/hr = 100 ml/750 mg x 60 mg/hr = **8 ml/hr**

97. 500 ml of D5W is to infuse in 6 hours. What is the drip rate?

   gtt/min = 60 gtt/ml x 83.3 ml/60 min = **83 gtt/min**
   **OR** gtt/min = 60 gtt/ml x 500 ml/360 min = 83.3 = **83 gtt/min**

98. You are to infuse 500 ml of D5NS at 130 ml/hr. What is the drip rate

   a. with 10 gtt/ml tubing?
   10 gtt/ml x 130 ml/60 min = **22 gtt/min**

   b. with 15 gtt/ml tubing?
   15 gtt/ml x 130 ml/60 min = **33 gtt/min**

c.   with 20 gtt/ml tubing?

20 gtt/ml x 130 ml/60 min = **43 gtt/min**

99.  Your medication is available 5 g (5000 mg) in 100 ml. You are to infuse it at 125 ml/hr. What is the hourly dosage?

mg/hr = 5000 mg/100 ml x 125 ml/hr = **6250 mg/hr**

100. The medication comes in a powdered form with 2 g in a vial. You add 8 ml of sterile water to reconstitute the medication. The MD has ordered 1200 mg of the medication be added to a 100 ml bag which is to be infused over 45 minutes.

a.   How much of the reconstituted medication will be added to the 100 ml bag?
ml = 8 ml/2000 mg x 1200 mg = **4.8 ml**

b.   What flow rate should you set to infuse the medication in 45 minutes?
ml/hr = 104.8 ml/45 min x 60 min/1 hr = **139.7 ml/hr**

101. Order reads 1000 ml D5 1/2 NS in 7 hours. Calculate flow rate and drip rate. The IV set is labeled 15 gtt/ml.

ml/hr = 1000 ml/7 hr = **142.9 ml/hr**
gtt/min = 15 gtt/ml x 142.9 ml/60 min = **36 gtt/min**

102. Order: 1500 ml NS to infuse at 90 ml/hr. The only tubing available is 20 gtt/ml.

a.   How long will it take to run in?
hr = 1 hr/90 ml x 1500 ml = 16.67 hr = **16 hr 40 min**

b.   What is the drip rate?
gtt/min = 20 gtt/ml x 90 ml/60 min = **30 gtt/min**

103. The order is for 1500 ml D5W. The drop factor is 15 gtt/ml, and the drip rate is 40 gtt/min. How many hours and minutes will it take to infuse?

min = 1 min/40 gtt x 15 gtt/ml x 1500 ml = 562.5 = 563 min = **9 hr 23 min**

104. Heparin is to infuse at 9 ml/hr. The IV solution is 25,000 units heparin in 250 ml D5W. What is the hourly dosage? What is the drip rate?

units/hr = 25,000 units/250 ml x 9 ml/hr = **900 units/hr**
gtt/min = 60 gtt/ml x 9 ml/60 min = **9 gtt/min**

105. The patient is to receive a heparin drip, concentration 10,000 units/100 ml D5W. It is to infuse at 7.6 ml/hr. What is the hourly dosage, and what is the gtt rate? The only tubing available is 10 gtt/ml.

units/hr = 10,000 units/100 ml x 7.6 ml/hr = **760 units/hr**
gtt/min = 10 gtt/ml x 7.6 ml/60 min = 1.3 = **1 gtt/min**

106. The order is to reconstitute Ancef to create a concentration of 1000 mg in 50 ml. It comes in a vial with 1 g in 2 ml. How much fluid must you add to reach the desired concentration? Then Ancef 1000 mg in 50 ml is to infuse over 45 minutes. What is the flow rate?

ml = 2 ml/1000 mg x 1000 mg = **2 ml**
ml/hr = 52 ml/45 min x 60 min/hr = **69.3 ml/hr**

107. The patient has acute gastroenteritis, and is on strict I&O. He is receiving LR 125 ml/hr, is getting Flagyl 1 g in 100 ml NS twice a day (infused over 60 minutes), and Ancef 1000 mg in 50 ml D5W every 8 hours (infused over 30 minutes). What is his 24-hour IV input?

| LR | | Flag | | Anc | | |
|---|---|---|---|---|---|---|
| 125 ml/hr | | 100 ml | | 50 ml | | |
| X 20.5 hr | | x 2 | | x 3 | | |
| 2562.5 | + | 200 ml | + | 150 ml | + | = **2912.5 ml** |
| | | - 2 hr | | - 1.5 hr | | |

108. D5W 2000 ml is to run for 16 hours. The only tubing available is 15 gtt/ml. What is the flow rate? The drip rate?

ml/hr = 2000 ml/16 hr = **125 ml/hr**
gtt/min = 15 gtt/ml x 125 ml/60 min = **31 gtt/min**


109. 500 ml 0.2NS is to infuse over 6 hours.

   a.   What tubing should you use?
        **Micro**, because the flow rate is less than 100 ml/hr

   b.   What is the drip rate?
        gtt/min = 60 gtt/ml x 500 ml/360 min = 83.3 = **83 gtt/min**

110. D5W 1800 ml is ordered, to infuse over 15 hours, using a 15 gtt/ml set. What are the flow rate and drip rate?

ml/hr = 1800 ml/15 hr = **120 ml/hr**
gtt/min = 15 gtt/ml x 120 ml/60 min = **30 gtt/min**


111. The order reads: Infuse 50 ml D5W in 40 minutes.

   a.   Tubing size?
        **Micro** because flow rate is less than 100 ml/hr

   b.   Flow rate?
        ml/hr = 50 ml/40 min x 60 min/hr = **75 ml/hr**

   c.   Drip rate?
        gtt/min = 60 gtt/ml x 75 ml/60 min = **75 gtt/min**

112. 1 L D5W is to infuse at 33 gtt/min using a 15 gtt/ml set. How long will it take to infuse?

min = 1 min/33 gtt x 15 gtt/ml x 1000 ml = 454.55 = 455 min = **7 hr 35 min**

113. Order: Transfuse 500 ml whole blood at 150 ml/hr. The transfusion was started at 1440.

   a.   How long will it take to infuse?
        hr = 1 hr/150 ml x 500 ml = 3.33 hr  = **3 hr 20 min**

   b.   What will be the completion time?
        **1800**

114. The MD orders 3500 ml D5.2NS to be given over the next 18 hours. Calculate the hourly and drip rate.

   ml/hr = 3500 ml/18 hr = **194.4 ml/hr**
   gtt/min = 10 gtt/ml x 194.4 ml/60 min = **32 gtt/min**

115. Levaquin 250 mg IV in 50 ml D5W is to be infused in one hour. What is the drip rate?

   gtt/min = 60 gtt/ml x 50 ml/60 min = **50 gtt/min**

116. An IV of 500 ml D5W is to infuse in 6 hours. The only tubing available is 10 gtt/ml. What is the drip rate?

   gtt/min = 10 gtt/ml x 83.3 ml/60 min = 13.9 = **14 gtt/min**

117. D5W 2000 ml is to run in 16 hours. The set calibration is 10 gtt/ml. What is the drip rate?

   gtt/min = 10 gtt/ml x 125 ml/60 min = 20.8 = **21 gtt/min**

118. LR at 80 ml/hr is hung. What is the drip rate, and how much fluid will the patient get over the next 24 hours?

   gtt/min = 60 gtt/ml x 80 ml/60 min = **80 gtt/min**
   ml = 80 ml/hr x 24 hr = **1920 ml**

119. Aminophylline 28 mg/hr is to be given to the patient IV. Available is aminophylline 500 mg in ½ L D5W. What is the hourly rate to be given, and what is the drip rate?

ml/hr = 500 ml/500 mg x 28 mg/hr = **28 ml/hr**
gtt/min = 60 gtt/ml x 28 ml/60 min = **28 gtt/min**

120. Cipro is available 1 g in a 2.6 ml vial. The doctor wants the patient to receive a 400 mg dose. How much fluid should you add to the 100 ml bag of D5W? Cipro 400 mg in 100 ml D5W is to infuse over 1 hour. Drip rate?

ml = 2.6 ml/1000 mg x 400 mg = 1.04 = **1 ml**
gtt/min = 10 gtt/ml x 101 ml/60 min = **17 gtt/min**

121. You are to give 1500 ml NS in 12 hours. Calculate the hourly and drip rate.

ml/hr = 1500 ml/12 hr = **125 ml/hr**
gtt/min = 10 gtt/ml x 125 ml/60 min = 20.8 = **21 gtt/min**

122. 1 liter of D5W is to infuse at 125 ml per hour. How long will it take to run in?

hr = 1 hr/125 ml x 1000 ml = **8 hr**

123. Aminophylline is ordered at 23 mg per hour. It is available 1 g in 500 ml of NS. What is the flow rate at which you will set the pump? What is the drip rate?

ml/hr = 500 ml/1000 mg x 23 mg/hr = **11.5 ml/hr**
gtt/min = 60 gtt/ml x 11.5 ml/60 min = 11.5 = **12 gtt/min**

124. Heparin has been mixed at 10,000 units in a 100 ml bag of NS. It is to infuse at 12 ml per hour. What is the hourly dosage?

units/hr = 10,000 units/100 ml x 12 ml/hr = **1200 units/hr**

125. 1 liter of D5 1/2 NS is to infuse over 12 hours. What is the flow rate? The drip rate? Tubing available: 15 gtt/ml.

ml/hr = 1000 ml/12 hr = **83.3 ml/hr**
gtt/min = 15 gtt/ml x 83.3 ml/60 min = 20.8 = **21 gtt/min**

126. You have been asked to keep input/output on a patient. He is NPO (getting nothing by mouth), but is on D5W at 125 ml/hr, and is also getting three antibiotics: Levaquin 250 mg in 100 ml (infused over 1 hour) daily, Keflex 500 mg in 250 ml (infused over 1 hour) three times a day, and Cipro 1 g in 150 ml (infused over 1 hour) twice a day. What is the total IV input in 24 hours?

| D5W | | Lev | | Kef | | Cip | |
|---|---|---|---|---|---|---|---|
| 125 ml/hr | | 100 ml | | 250 ml | | 150 ml | |
| X 18 hr | | x 1 | | x 3 | | x 2 | |
| 2250 ml | + | 100 ml | + | 750 ml | + | 300 ml | = **3400 ml** |
| | | - 1 hr | | - 3 hr | | - 2 hr | |

127. The dehydrated patient is to get 500 ml over the next 90 minutes. At what rate will you set the pump?

ml/hr = 500 ml/90 min x 60 min/1 hr = **333.3 ml/hr**

128. The doctor has ordered 2 liters of LR to be given to the patient during the next 15 hours. What is the drip rate?

ml/hr = 2000 ml/15 hr = 133.3 ml/hr
gtt/min = 10 gtt/ml x 133.3 ml/60 min = **22 gtt/min**

129. There are 380 ml left in the IV bag. It is now 1400. The patient has a test scheduled at 1700. At what rate should you set the pump to be sure the infusion is complete before the test?

ml/hr = 380 ml/3 hr = **126.7 ml/hr**

130. 250 ml of NS was started at 0900, infusing at 48 gtt/min and using 15 gtt/ml tubing. How long will it take to infuse? What will the flow rate be?

min = 1 min/48 gtt x 15 gtt/ml x 250 ml = 78 min = **1 hr 18 min**
ml/hr = 1 ml/15 gtt x 48 gtt/min x 60 min/hr = **192 ml/hr**

131. Calculate the drip rate for 50 ml of Ancef to infuse over 30 minutes. Then calculate the drip rate for 100 ml of Zithromycin to infuse over 60 minutes.

gtt/min = 10 gtt/ml x 50 ml/30 min = **17 gtt/min**
gtt/min = 10 gtt/ml x 100 ml/60 min = **17 gtt/min**

132. 750 ml of D5LR is running at 40 gtt/min with a 15 gtt/ml tubing set. What is its infusion rate? How long will it take to finish running?

ml/hr = 1 ml/15 gtt x 40 gtt/min x 60 min/hr = **160 ml/hr**
min = 1 min/40 gtt x 15 gtt/ml x 750 ml = 281 min **= 4 hr 41 min**
**OR** hr = 1 hr/160 ml x 750 ml = 4.69 hr = **4 hr 41 min**

133. 500 mg of Zosyn in 100 ml NS is to infuse at 60 mg per hour. What is the flow rate? The drip rate?

ml/hr = 100 ml/500 mg x 60 mg/hr = **12 ml/hr**
gtt/min = 60 gtt/ml x 12 ml/60 min = **12 gtt/min**

134. Using IV tubing with a drop factor of 15 gtt/ml, and an order for 250 ml NS to be given over 8 hours, calculate the flow rate and drip rate.

ml/hr = 250 ml/8 hr = **31.3 ml/hr**
gtt/min = 15 gtt/ml x 31.3 ml/hr = 7.8 = **8 gtt/min**

135. 50 ml of an antibiotic is to be infused in 20 minutes. What is the flow rate? What tubing size will you use?

ml/hr = 50 ml/20 min x 60 min/hr = **150 ml/hr**

**Will use macro tubing**

136. The patient has an oncology drug prescribed. The doctor orders 15 mg/kg/day, in four divided doses. The patient weighs 157 pounds. How much will the patient receive per dose?

mg = 15 mg/Kg x 1 Kg/2.2 lb x 157 lb = 1070.5 mg per day
    per day
mg/dose = 1070.5 mg/day x 1 day/4 doses = **267.6 mg/dose**

137. If a medication comes 500 mg/250 ml, and each dose is to infuse in 45 minutes, what flow rate will you set for each dose?

ml/hr = 250 ml/45 min x 60 min/hr = **333.3 ml/hr**

138. The doctor has ordered the dehydrated patient to receive 3 liters of LR in the next 16 hours. Calculate the flow rate and drip rate.

ml/hr = 3000 ml/16 hr = **187.5 ml/hr**
gtt min = 10 gtt/ml x 187.5 ml/60 min = **31 gtt/min**

139. Your patient has a 500 ml bolus of NS to be infused at 125 ml/hr. How long will it take to infuse?

hr = 1 hr/125 ml x 500 ml = **4 hr**

140. Calculate the drip rate of 1 liter of D5 1/2 NS infusing at 140 ml/hr, using:

    a.    10 gtt/ml tubing
           gtt/min = 10 gtt/ml x 140 ml/60 min = **23 gtt/min**

   b.    15 gtt/ml tubing
         gtt min = 15 gtt/ml x 140 ml/60 min = **35 gtt/min**

   c.    20 gtt/ml tubing
         gtt/min = 20 gtt/ml x 140 ml/60 min = **47 gtt/min**

141.  The flow rate of your patient's medication is 160 ml/hr. What is the drip rate?

      gtt/min = 10 gtt/ml x 160 ml/60 min = **27 gtt/min**

142.  Available: 3 g in 2 ml NS, to be added to a 100 ml bag of NS

      Order: Give at 700 mg/hr
      Flow rate?
      ml/hr = 102 ml/3000 mg x 700 mg/hr = 71,400/3,000 = **23.8 ml/hr**

143.  The medication comes in a 10 ml vial containing 0.5 g/ml. The doctor has ordered 2 g in 100 ml D5W.

   a.    How much medication will you add to the bag?
         ml = 1 ml/0.5 g x 2 g = **4 ml**

   b.    What flow rate will you set to infuse it in 30 minutes?
         ml/hr = 104 ml/30 min x 60 min/hr = **208 ml/hr**

144.  The ordered medication is available 250 mg/ml. You are to give 2 g in a 100 ml bag of D5NS. What rate would you set on the pump to infuse it in 45 minutes?

      ml = 1 ml/250 mg x 2000 mg = 8 ml
      ml/hr = 108 ml/45 min x 60 min/hr = **144 ml/hhr**

      **Note that you <u>must</u> do this problem in two steps for the correct answer.**

145. You hang 250 ml of medicine at 0900, using 15 gtt/ml tubing and a drip rate of 26 gtt/min. At what time will the bag be empty?

min = 1 min/26 gtt x 15 gtt/ml x 250 ml = 144 min = 2 hr 24 min
So the bag will be empty at **1124**.

146. Heparin 25,000 units in 250 ml NS is infusing at 13.7 ml/hr. Calculate the drip rate.

gtt/min = 60 gtt/ml x 13.7 ml/60 min = 13.7 = **14 gtt/min**

147. 500 ml of NS is infusing at 35 gtt/min using 20 gtt/ml tubing. Calculate the flow rate.

ml/hr = 1 ml/20 gtt x 35 gtt/min x 60 min/hr = **105 ml/hr**

148. You add 8 ml of sterile water to reconstitute 2 g of a powdered medication. The doctor's order is to give 1.5 g of the medication in 100 ml of NS over 1 hour.

a. How much fluid will you add to the 100 ml bag?
ml = 8 ml/2 g x 1.5 g = **6 ml**

b. What flow rate will you set to infuse the medication?
ml/hr = **106 ml/hr** No calculations are necessary, since time is 1 hr.

149. 30 mEq of potassium in 100 ml 0.45NS is infusing over 90 minutes. What is the hourly dosage?

mEq/hr = 30 mEq/90 min x 60 min/hr = **20 mEq/hr**

150. Your patient is to receive a medication at 12 mg/Kg, which is to be added to a 100 ml bag of NS and to infuse at 38 mg/hr. The patient weighs 118.8 lb. Calculate the flow rate.

mg = 12 mg/Kg x 1 Kg/2.2 lb x 118.8 lb = 648 mg
ml/hr = 100 ml/648 mg x 38 mg/hr = **5.9 ml/hr**

# PEDIATRIC DOSAGE CALCULATIONS

1. Your patient weighs 11.4 Kg. According to the literature, the safe dose is 25 to 40 mg/Kg/day in four divided doses. The doctor has ordered 100 mg per dose. Is his order safe?

   mg = 25 mg/Kg x 11.4 Kg = 285 mg/day 285mg/4 doses = 71.25 mg/dose
   mg = 40 mg/Kg x 11.4 Kg = 456 mg/day; 456 mg/4 doses = 114 mg/dose
   **Yes, the order is safe; it falls within the safe range.**

2. Your source indicates the safe range is 20 – 30 mg/Kg/day in two divided doses. The medication is available 50 mg/ml. The doctor has ordered 75 mg per dose. The patient weighs 18 lb.

   a. Is the doctor's order safe?
      mg = 20 mg/Kg x 8.18 Kg = 163.6 mg/day; 163.6mg/2 doses = 81.8 mg/dose
      mg = 30 mg/Kg x 8.18 Kg = 245.4 mg/day; 245.4 mg/2 doses = 122.7 mg/dose
      **No, the order is not safe; it is outside the safe range.**

   b. How much would you give, in ml, according to the doctor's order?
      ml = 1 ml/50 mg x 75 mg = **1.5 ml**

3. The doctor has ordered maintenance fluids on your 27.82 Kg pediatric patient. At what rate will you set the pump to give these fluids over the next 24 hours?

   | 100 | x | 10 | = | 1000 ml |
   |-----|---|------|---|---------|
   | 50 | x | 10 | = | 500 ml |
   | 20 | x | 7.82 | = | 156.4 ml |
   | | | | | 1656.4 ml |

   1656.4 ml/24 hr = **69.02 ml/hr**

4. The child is to receive 20 mg of a medication per dose, by MD order. Your source states the medication is safe at 50 mg/day in three divided doses. What is the safe dose? And is the doctor's order safe?

   mg/dose = 50 mg/day x 1 day/3 doses = 16.67 mg/dose

   **Safe dose is 16.67 mg, so doctor's order is not safe.**

5.  What is the $M^2$ for a child who weighs 22.4 Kg and is 50.8 cm tall?

    $M^2 = \sqrt{\underline{22.4 \times 50.8}/3600} = \sqrt{0.31609} = \mathbf{0.56\ M^2}$

6.  The doctor has ordered 1.5 x maintenance fluids for a child weighing 41.6 Kg.

    a.  How much fluid will the child get in 24 hours?
        100 ml/Kg x 10 Kg = 1000 ml
        50 ml/Kg x 10 Kg = 500 ml
        20 ml/Kg x 21.6 Kg = 432 ml
        1000 + 500 + 432 = 1932 ml x 1.5 = **2898 ml**

    b.  Given over a 24-hour period, at what rate would you set the pump to infuse this fluid?
        ml/hr = 2898 ml/24 hr = **120.75 ml/hr**

7.  Your 4-year-old, 35 lb. dehydrated patient has a bolus dose of 500 ml of NS to be infused over 4 hours, after which he is to receive 0.45NS at 3.8 ml/Kg/hr.

    a.  What hourly rate will you set for the bolus dose?
        ml/hr = 500 ml/4 hr = **125 ml/hr**

    b.  At what rate will the 0.45NS infuse?
        ml/hr = 3.8 ml/Kg x 15.91 Kg = **60.46 ml/hr**

8.  Your patient has D5NS infusing at 45 ml/hr. She also has an NG tube, which has drained 110 ml in the previous 12-hour shift. The doctor has ordered D5NS NG replacement fluids. At what rate should you set the pump to comply with the doctor's orders?

    ml/hr = 110 ml/12 hr = 9.17 ml/hr

    **Reset pump to 45 ml/hr + 9.17 ml/hr = 54.17 ml/hr**

9. What is the $M^2$ for a child who is 33 inches tall and weighs 42 lb?

cm = 2.54 cm/in x 33 in = 83.82 cm
Kg = 1 Kg/2.2 lb x 42 lb = 19.09 Kg

$M^2 = \sqrt{19.09 \times 83.82}/3600 = \sqrt{0.44448} = \mathbf{0.67\ M^2}$

10. The literature indicates a safe dose of a medication is 12 to 35 mg/$M^2$. For the patient in problem 9, the doctor has ordered 60 mg/day in six divided doses. Is his order safe?

mg = 12 mg/$M^2$ x 0.67 $M^2$ = 8.04 mg/dose or 48.24 mg/day
mg = 35 mg/$M^2$ x 0.67 $M^2$ = 23.45 mg/dose or 140.7/day

**Doctor's order is 10 mg/dose or 60 mg/day; it is safe.**

11. Your source states the medication's safe dose is 3.5 mg/Kg. Your patient weighs 69 lb. The doctor has ordered 120 mg. Is the order safe?

mg = 3.5 mg/Kg x 1 Kg/2.2 lb x 69 lb = 109.77 mg

**The doctor's order is not safe.**

12. Your patient's NG tube drained 138 ml during the previous shift. The patient has ½ NS infusing at 30 ml/hr. The doctor has ordered D5 1/2 NS replacement fluids. At what rate will you set the pump to replace the fluid lost to the NG tube?

ml/hr = 138 ml/12 hours = **11.5 ml/hr** (2 different fluids require 2 different pumps)

13. A medication has been ordered for an infant at 3 mg/Kg. The child weighs 5 lb 7 oz. How much will you give?

5 lb 7 oz = 5 lb + 7/16 lb = 5.4375 lb; Kg = 1 Kg/2.2 lb x 5.4375 lb = 2.47 Kg
mg = 3 mg/Kg x 2.47 Kg = **7.41 mg**

14. A medication is cited in the literature as being safe at 8 – 20 mg/M². Your patient's M² is 0.98. What is the maximum dose you could safely give?

    mg = 20 mg/M² x 0.98 M² = **19.6 mg**

15. The doctor has ordered maintenance fluids under the 100-50-20 protocol for a child weighing 49 Kg. How much fluid will the child receive over the next 24 hours, per the doctor's order?

    | 100 ml/Kg | x | 10 Kg | = | 1000 ml |
    |---|---|---|---|---|
    | 50 ml/Kg | x | 10 Kg | = | 500 ml |
    | 20 ml/Kg | x | 29 Kg | = | 580 ml |
    | 1000 + 500 + 580 | | | = | **2080 ml** |

16. The dehydrated teenager is to receive a one-liter bolus of D5NS over 6 hours, and then to continue D5NS at 125 ml/hr. How much IV fluid will he receive in the next 24 hours?

    1000 ml over 1st six hours
    2250 ml over next 18 hours (125 ml/hr x 18 hr = 2250)
    **Total of 3250 ml over the next 24 hours.**

17. The child weighs 13.6 Kg. The medication is to be given at 20 – 30 mg/Kg/day in four divided doses. What is the safe range per dose?

    mg = 20 mg/Kg x 13.6 Kg = 272 mg/day; 272 mg/4 doses = 68 mg/dose
    mg = 30 mg/Kg x 13.6 Kg = 408 mg/day; 408 mg/4 doses = 102 mg/dose
    Safe range is **68 to 102 mg/dose.**

18. The medication is available in vials with a concentration of 300 mg/5 ml. You are to dilute 175 mg of the medication in a 100 ml bag of D5W. How much of the medication will you add to the bag?

    ml = 5 ml/300 mg x 175 mg = **2.92 ml**

19. For the previous problem, at what rate would you set the pump if the child weighs 1.59 Kg and is to receive 2 mg/Kg/min. of the medication?

mg/hr = 2 mg/Kg x 1.59 Kg = 3.18 mg/min x 60 min/hr = 190.8 mg/hr
ml/hr = 102.92 ml/175 mg x 190.8 mg/hr = **112.21 ml/hr**

$$\frac{102.92\,ml}{175\,mg} \times \frac{190.8\,mg}{1\,hr}$$

20. Calculate the $M^2$ for a patient who weighs 28.7 Kg and is 34.3 cm tall.

$M^2 = \sqrt{28.7 \times 34.3/3600} = \sqrt{0.27345} = $ **0.52 $M^2$**

21. If the recommended child's dose is 4 – 12 mg/$M^2$, what is the safe dose range for the patient whose $M^2$ you just calculated in problem 20?

mg = 4 mg/$M^2$ x 0.52 $M^2$ = 2.08 mg
mg = 12 mg/$M^2$ x 0.52 $M^2$ = 6.24 mg

**Safe range is 2.08 to 6.24 mg.**

22. The doctor has ordered 1.5 x maintenance fluids for a child weighing 39.8 Kg. At what rate would you set a pump to infuse these fluids over 24 hours?

| | | | |
|---|---|---|---|
| 100 ml/Kg | x | 10 Kg | = | 1000 ml |
| 50 ml/Kg | x | 10 Kg | = | 500 m l |
| 20 ml/Kg | x | 19.8 Kg | = | 396 ml |
| 1000 + 500 + 396 | | | = | 1896 ml x 1.5 = 2844 ml |

ml/hr = 2844 ml/24 hr = **118.5 ml/hr**

23. Your 8-year-old post-surgical patient has an NG tube which drained 231 ml during the previous shift. The patient has D5 1/2 NS infusing at 35 ml/hr. The doctor has ordered D5 1/2 NS as replacement fluid. At what rate will you set the pump to infuse the lost fluid over the next 12 hours?

Ml/hr = 231ml/12 hr = 19.25 ml/hr
35 ml/hr + 19.25 ml/hr = **54.25 ml/hr** because the replacement fluids are
the same as the current fluids

24. The order is for 300 mg every 6 hours. The patient weighs 43.7 Kg. The safe range in the literature is 20 – 50 mg/Kg/day in three divided doses. Is the order safe?

mg = 20 mg/Kg x 43.7 Kg = 874 mg/day; 874 mg/3 doses = 291.33 mg/dose
mg = 50 mg/Kg x 43.7 Kg = 2185 mg/day; 2185 mg/3 doses = 728.33 mg/dose

**Doctor's order is 300 mg/dose, 1200 mg/day, so it is safe.**
Even though he has ordered four doses a day rather than three per the literature, both his per dose and per day orders are within the safe ranges.

25. The doctor has ordered 50 mg of a medication for the child. Your patient weighs 12.3 Kg. The literature states the medication is safe at 6 mg/Kg.

   a. What is the safe dose for this child?
   mg = 6 mg/Kg x 12.3 Kg = **73.8 mg**

   b. Is the doctor's order safe?

   **No, the doctor's order is not safe – is below the safe dose.**

26. The order is for 5.8 mg/Kg/day in three divided doses. Your patient weighs 18.2 Kg, and the medication comes 150 mg/50 ml. How many ml will the child receive per dose?

mg = 5.8 mg/Kg x 18.2 Kg = 105.56 mg/day
105.56 mg/day x 1 day/3 doses = 35.19 mg/dose
ml = 50 ml/150 mg x 35.19 mg = **11.73 ml**

27. Post-surgery, your three-year-old patient has an NG tube with drainage of 173 ml during the last shift. He has D5LR running at 60 ml/hr. The doctor orders replacement fluids of D5.45NS with 10 mEq of KCl which (after some quick calculations with the NG output) he orders to run at 74.4 ml/hr. Is he correct? If not, why not?

**No, he is incorrect. Although the replacement fluids will run in at 14.42 ml/hr, they cannot simply be added to the current IV fluids, because they are different from the current fluid, and must therefore infuse separately and into a separate site, using a separate pump.**

28. Your 34 lb patient is to receive 150 mg of a medication every six hours. The safe range is 25 – 50 mg/Kg/day in divided doses. Is the order a safe dose for the child?

mg = 25 mg/Kg x 15.45 Kg = 386.25 mg/day; 386.25/4 = 96.56 mg/dose
mg = 50 mg/Kg x 15.45 Kg = 772.5 mg/day; 772.5/4 = 193.13 mg/dose

**MD has ordered 150 mg/dose (safe), which is 600 mg/day (also safe).**
Note that the literature does not specify the number of doses. Therefore, to determine a safe dose, we use the number of doses the doctor has ordered to do our calculations.

29. The doctor has ordered twice maintenance fluids for your 27 Kg patient. After calculating, he orders them to run at 68.3 ml/hr for the next 24 hours. Are his calculations correct?

100 ml/Kg x 10 Kg = 1000 ml
50 ml/Kg x 10 Kg = 500 ml
20 ml/Kg x 7 Kg = 140 ml
1000 + 500 + 140 = 1640 x 2 = 3280 ml
3280ml/24 hr = 136.67 ml/hr.
**He is incorrect. He has calculated based on maintenance fluids, not the *twice* maintenance fluids he ordered.**

30. Referenced pediatric dosage is 25 mg/kg day. What is a safe daily dose for your newborn 6.36 Kg patient?

**mg = 25 mg/Kg x 6.36 Kg = 159 mg**

31. What is the M$^2$ for a patient who is 4 ft. 10 in. and 102 lb?

cm = 2.54 cm/1 in x 58 in = 147.32 cm
Kg = 1 Kg/2.2 lb x 102 lb = 46.36 Kg

M$^2$ = $\sqrt{147.32 \times 46.36/3600}$ = $\sqrt{1.89715}$ = **1.38 M$^2$**

32. The literature states the safe range for the medication is 18 – 25 mg/M² per day in two divided doses. Using the M² from problem 31, what is the safe range per dose?

$$Mg = 18 \text{ mg/M}^2 \times 1.38 \text{ M}^2 = 24.84 \text{ mg/2} = \textbf{12.42 mg}$$
per day            per day      **per dose**
25 mg/M² x 1.38 M²     34.5 mg/2 = **17.25 mg**

33. For the patient in problem 31, another medication is to be given at 30 mg per M² per day. What daily dose should the patient receive of this medication?

mg = 30 mg/M² x 1.38 M² = **41.4 mg**

34. The child has IV fluids infusing at 40 ml/hr. The doctor has ordered a 500 ml bolus to be given over six hours, to be added to the current IV fluids. At what rate will you set the pump during that six-hour period?

ml/hr = 500 ml/6 hr = 83.33 ml/hr + 40 ml/hr = **123.33 ml/hr**

35. The baby weighs 8 lb 13 oz. The safe dose of the medication order is 40 mg/Kg/day in three divided doses. What is the safe dose per day for this child? Safe dose per dose?

Kg = 1 Kg/2.2 lb x 8.8125 lb = 4.01 Kg

**Daily** safe dose: 40 mg/Kg x 4.01 Kg = **160.4 mg**

**Per dose:** 160.4 mg/day x 1 day/3 doses = **53.47 mg**

36. Your 18-month-old patient has lost 106 ml in NG drainage in the past 12 hours. What flow rate will you set for the child's replacement fluids?

ml/hr = 106 ml/12 hr = **8.83 ml/hr**

37. The order is for 300 mg of an antibiotic to be given in 100 ml of D5.45NS over 40 minutes three times daily. Your reference indicates a safe dose is 20 – 40 mg/Kg/day in two divided doses. Your patient weighs 30 Kg.

   a. Is the order safe?

   20 mg/Kg x 30 Kg = 600 mg/day or 300 mg/dose
   40 mg/Kg x 30 Kg = 1200 mg/day or 600 mg/dose
   **The order is safe.** It is safe per dose at 300 mg/dose, and safe per day at 900 mg/day. Even though the doctor ordered three doses per day instead of the two indicated in the reference, the ordered amounts still fall within the safe ranges, both per dose and per day.

   b. At what rate will you set the pump?

   ml/hr = 100 ml/40 min x 60 min/hr = **150 ml/hr**

38. Your patient is 48 cm tall and weighs 9.2 Kg. The medication is ordered at 125 mg/M². How much will the child receive?

   $M^2 = \sqrt{48 \times 9.2/3600} = \sqrt{0.12267} = 0.35\ M^2$
   mg = 125 mg/M² x 0.35 M² = **43.75 mg**

39. According to the literature, the safe range for the medication is 8 – 20 mg/Kg/day in four divided doses. What is the minimum safe dose for your 18.3 Kg patient?

   mg = 8 mg/Kg x 18.3 Kg = 146.4 mg/day
   mg = 146.4 mg/day x 1 day/4 doses = **36.6 mg**

40. D5NS is infusing into your patient at 45 ml/hr. She has an NG tube through which she has lost 180 ml in the previous shift. The doctor has ordered NS with 10 mEq KCl as replacement fluids. At what rate will the replacement fluids infuse?

   ml/hr = 180 ml/12 hr = **15 ml/hr**
   The fluids are different, so must infuse on different pumps.

41.  Your 23.68 Kg patient has maintenance fluids ordered, to be given over the next 12 hours. At what rate will you set the pump?

| 100 x 10 | = | 1000 ml | ml/hr = 1573.6ml/12 hr = **131.13 ml/hr** |
| 50 x 10 | = | 500 ml | |
| 20 x 3.68 | = | 73.6 ml | |
| | | 1573.6 ml | |

42.  The medication is available 0.75 mg/ml. The order is for 60 mcg/Kg for your 71.4 lb patient. How many ml will you give?

Kg = 1 Kg/2.2 lb x 71.4 lb = 32.45 Kg

ml = 1 ml/0.75 mg x 1 mg/1000 mcg x 60 mcg/1 Kg x 32.45 Kg = 1947/750 = **2.6 ml**

43.  The literature gives a safe range of 20 – 50 mg/Kg/day in four divided doses. The doctor has ordered 100 mg every four hours. The child weighs 19 Kg. Is the doctor's order safe?

20 mg/Kg x 19 Kg = 380 mg/day over 4 doses = 95 mg/dose
50 mg/Kg x 19 Kg = 950 mg/day over 4 doses = 237.5 mg/dose
**The doctor's order is safe, both per dose and per day. Although he has ordered more doses per day than the literature indicates, his ordered dose still falls within safe parameters both per dose (100 mg ordered) and per day (600 mg ordered).**

44.  Your 27.3 Kg patient is put on half maintenance. At what rate will you set the IV pump to deliver the fluids?

100 ml/Kg x 10 Kg = 1000 ml
50 ml/Kg x 10 Kg = 500 ml
20 ml/Kg x 7.3 Kg = 146 ml

1000 + 500 + 146 = 1646 ml/2 = 823 ml per the MD's half maintenance order

ml/hr = 823 ml/24 hr = **34.29 ml/hr**

45. Your patient has NS infusing at 30 ml/hr. The doctor orders a 500 ml bolus dose to infuse over the next 4 hours. The infusion rate will then revert to its pre-bolus rate. How much fluid will the patient receive over the next 24 hours?

    125 ml/hr x 4 hr = 500 ml (the bolus)
    30 ml/hr x 20 hr = 600 ml for a total of **1100 ml**

46. The child is to receive 40 mcg/Kg/min. of the medication ordered. The medication is available 1 g in 250 ml. The patient weighs 29.8 Kg. How many mg will the patient receive per hour?

    $$mg = 1\ mg/1000\ mcg \times \frac{40\ mcg/Kg}{per\ min.} \times 29.8\ Kg = 1.192\ mg/minute$$
    1.192 mg/min x 60 min/hr = **71.52 mg/hr**

47. In the previous problem, at what rate would you set the pump for the calculated dose to infuse?

    ml/hr = 250 ml/1000 mg x 71.52 mg/hr = **17.88 ml/hr**

48. Your 73 lb patient has a medication ordered at 100 mg per dose. The safe range, per the pharmacy, is 10 – 25 mg/Kg/day in four divided doses. Is the doctor's order safe?

    mg = 10 mg/Kg x 33.18 Kg = 331.8 mg/day = 82.95 mg/dose
    mg = 25 mg/Kg x 33.18 Kg = 829.5 mg/day = 207.38 mg/dose

    **Yes, the order is safe.**

49. The medication is available at 125 mg/10 ml. The safe dose is 15 – 25 mg/Kg/day in three divided doses. Your patient weighs 22.7 Kg. The doctor has ordered 15 ml per dose. Is the order safe?

    mg = 15 mg/Kg x 22.7 Kg = 340.5 mg/day = 113.5 mg/dose
    mg = 25 mg/Kg x 22.7 Kg = 567.5 mg/day = 189.17 mg/dose

    **MD has ordered mg = 125 mg/10 ml x 15 ml = 187.5 mg per dose; order is safe.**

50. Available: 500 mg/10 ml in 10 ml vials
    Order: 175 mg in 50 ml of ½ NS

    a.  How much of the available medication should be added to the NS?
        ml = 10 ml/500 mg x 175 mg = **3.5 ml**

    b.  At what rate will you set the pump for this medication to infuse in 30 minutes?
        ml/hr = 53.5 ml/30 min x 60 min/1 hr = **107 ml/hr**

    c.  The doctor has ordered the child should not receive IV fluids at more than 12 ml/hr/Kg. The child weighs 7.8 Kg. Will you need to call the doctor to question the order?

    **Yes**. Maximum flow rate the doctor wants to permit is 12 ml/hr per Kg x 7.8 Kg = 93.6 ml/hr. The doctor may change his order, or retain the order but expand the time for infusion. For example, if the infusion time was expanded to 45 minutes, the flow rate would be
    53.5 ml/45 min x 60 min/hr = 71.3 ml/hr, within his guidelines

51. The doctor has ordered 150 mg of a medication three times daily for your pediatric patient, who weighs 27.8 Kg. The usual dose is 5 to 20 mg/Kg/day in divided doses. Is the doctor's order safe?

    5 mg/Kg x 27.8 Kg = 139 mg/day = 46.33 mg/dose
    Per day
    20 mg/Kg x 27.8 Kg = 556 mg/day = 185.33 mg/dose

    The doctor has ordered 450 mg/day, 150 mg/dose. Both fall within the safe ranges, so **the order is safe.**

52. According to the literature, the medication's usual dose is 25 to 40 mg/Kg/day in divided doses. What is the safe range for your 29.6 lb patient?

    25 mg/Kg x 1 Kg/2.2 lb x 29.6 lb = **336.36 mg**
    Per day                                       to      per day
    40 mg/Kg x 1 Kg/2.2 lb x 29.6 lb = **538.18 mg**

53. The child is to receive a medication at 2.5 mcg/Kg/min. The child weighs 23.6 Kg. What is the hourly dosage in mg/hr?

mg/hr = 1 mg/1000 mcg x $\dfrac{2.5 \text{ mcg/Kg}}{\text{per min.}}$ x 23.6 Kg = 0.059 mg/min x 60 min/1 hr = **3.54 mg/hr**

54. Calculate the M² of a child weighing 11 lb 6 oz. and 23 in. long.

M² = √ 5.17 x 58.42 / 3600 = √ 0.0839 = **0.29 M²**

55. The recommended dose is 30 mg/M² to 50 mg/M². What is the safe range for your patient in problem 54?

mg = 30 mg/M² x 0.29 M² = **8.7 mg**

**to**

mg = 50 mg/M² x 0.29 M² = **14.5 mg**

56. The child has D5W NG replacement fluids ordered for the 146 ml of fluid lost to the NG in the prior shift. He is also to receive 1.5x maintenance fluids over the next 24 hours. The child weighs 22.46 Kg. What rate will you set for each fluid?

NG repl. fluid 146 ml/12 hr =     **12.17 ml/hr**

Maint. fluid   100 x 10   =   1000 ml
               50 x 10    =   500 ml
               20 x 2.46  =   49.2 ml
                               1549.2 x 1.5 = 2323.8 ml/24 hr = **96.83 ml/hr**

57. The order is for 450 mg of a medication every 8 hours. The safe dose per your reference is 60 – 90 mg/Kg/day. The drug is available 125 mg/ml. Your patient weighs 22.3 Kg.

   a.  What is the safe range for your patient?
       60 mg/Kg x 22.3 Kg = **1338 mg/day** divided by 3 = **446 mg/dose**
       Per day                          to                              to
       90 mg/Kg x 22.3 Kg = **2007 mg/day** divided by 3 = **669 mg/dose**

b.    Is the doctor's order safe?
      450 mg/8 hr x 24 hr/1 day = 1350 mg **Yes, both per dose & per day.**

c.    How much of the medication will the child receive per dose in ml?
      ml = 1 ml/125 mg x 450 mg = **3.6 ml**

58.  The doctor determines your pediatric patient is slightly dehydrated, and orders a 500 ml bolus of D5W to be infused over the next 8 hours. The child currently has D5W infusing at 40 ml/hr. What rate will you need to set for the next 8 hours to give the ordered bolus?

500 ml/8 hr = 62.5 ml for the bolus + 40 ml/hr already infusing = **102.5 ml/hr for the next 8 hours**.

After the bolus finishes infusing, the flow rate will revert to 40 ml/hr.

59.  Your patient weighs 14.7 Kg. Your reference states the safe dose for a medication ordered is 40 to 70 mg/kg/day in four divided doses. The doctor has ordered 200 mg every four hours.

a.    What is the safe range?
      mg = 40 mg/Kg x 14.7 Kg = **588 mg/day** divided by 4 doses = **147 mg/dose**
           per day                              to                                    to
      mg = 70 mg/Kg x 14.7 Kg = **1029 mg/day** divided by 4 doses = **257.25 mg/dose**

b.    Is the doctor's order safe?

      **No.** It is safe per dose, but he has ordered 6 doses/day or 1200 mg/day, above the safe per day range, so his **order is unsafe**.
      Remember: in verifying the safety of the doctor's order, be sure to always check it against <u>both</u> the per day <u>and</u> the per dose safe ranges.

60.  Calculate the M² for a pediatric patient who is 55 cm tall and weighs 13.7 Kg.

$M^2 = \sqrt{55 \times 13.7/3600} = \sqrt{0.20931} =$ **0.46 M²**

61. Using the M² calculated in problem 60, what is the safe dose for a medication to be given at 20 mg/M²?

    mg = 20 mg/M² x 0.46 M² = **9.2 mg**

62. A child is to receive 150 mg of a medication. The medication is available 750 mg of powder in a 10 ml vial. You are to add enough fluid to the vial to create a 200 mg/ml concentration.

    a. How much fluid will you add to the vial to create the desired concentration?
    Ml = 1 ml/200 mg x 750 mg = **3.75 ml**

    b. How much will you give your patient, in ml?
    Ml = 1 ml/200 mg x 150 mg = **0.75 ml**

63. Your patient weighs 38.6 Kg. The doctor has ordered 1.5 x maintenance fluids per the usual 100-50-20 rule. How much IV fluid will your patient receive in the next 24 hours as maintenance fluids?

    100 ml/Kg x 10 Kg    =    1000 ml
    50 ml/Kg x 10 Kg     =    500 ml
    20 ml/kg x 18.6 Kg   =    372 ml
                              1872 x 1.5 = **2808 ml**

64. What is the M² for a newborn who weighs 8 lb 10 oz and is 22 inches long?

    cm = 2.54 cm/in x 22 in = 55.88 cm; 8 lb 10 oz = 8.625 lb; Kg = 1 Kg/2.2 lb x 8.625 lb = 3.92 Kg

    M² = √ 55.88 x 3.92/3600 = √ 0.06085 = **0.25 M²**

65. Your pediatric patient has an NG tube, with 78 ml of output in the past 12 hours. He has D5NS infusing at 40 ml/hr. The MD has ordered NG replacement fluids of D5NS with 10 mEq KCl. At what rate would you set the pump to replace the fluids lost through the NG tube?

    Ml/hr = 78ml/12 hr = **6.5 ml/hr**
    Again, the two fluids are not the same: the potassium in the replacement fluid is absent

in the fluid already infusing. To add the two amounts together, the two fluids must be <u>identical.</u>

66. The literature states the safe dosage range for the ordered medication is 40-70 mg/Kg/dose, not to exceed 6 g per day. Your patient weighs 37.2 Kg.

   a.   What is the safe range for your patient?

   40 mg/Kg x 37.2 Kg =        **1488 mg**
   Per dose                            **to**              per dose
   70 g/Kg x 37.2 Kg    =     **2604 mg**

   b.   The doctor ordered 2 g every 8 hours. Is his order safe?

   **Yes.** It falls within the per dose range just calculated, and does not exceed the daily maximum, so is safe.

67. The doctor ordered the medication at 5 mg/Kg/day in four doses for your 42 Kg patient. The medication is available only in 10 ml vials containing 250 mg of the medication. How many ml will your patient receive per dose?

   mg = 5 mg/Kg x 42 Kg = 210 mg/day x 1 day/4 doses = 52.5 mg/dose
   ml/dose = 10 ml/250 mg x 52.5 mg/dose = **2.1 ml**

68. Calculate the safe dose per day for a 29.7 lb patient for a medication ordered at 7.5 mg/Kg/day.

   mg      =      7.5 mg/Kg x 1 Kg/2.2 lb x 29.7 lb = **101.25 mg/day**
                         per day

69. The child is to get a bolus dose of 500 ml of D51/2 NS, infused over a four-hour period. At what rate will it infuse?

   500 ml/4 hr = **125 ml/hr**

70. The neonate, who weighs 8 lb. 3 oz., is to receive 2x maintenance fluids. At what rate will they infuse over the next 24 hours?

8 lb 3 oz = 8 lb 3/16 lb = 8.1875 lb = 3.72 Kg
100 x 3.72 = 372 ml x 2 = 744 ml/24 hr = **31 ml/hr**

71. The child has lost 130 ml through an NG tube. The fluid is to be replaced with D5NS during your 12-hour shift. The child currently has D5NS infusing at 45 ml/hr. At what rate will you set the pump to replace the lost fluid?

ml/hr = 130 ml/12 hr = 10.8 ml/hr + 45 ml/hr now infusing = **55.83 ml/hr for the next 12 hours**

72. The doctor ordered ½ maintenance fluids for your 73-lb patient.

    a.    How much fluid will the patient receive in the next 24 hours?

Kg = 1 Kg/2.2 lb x 73 lb = 33.18 Kg

| 100 ml/Kg | x 10 Kg | = | 1000 ml |
| 50 ml/Kg | x 10 Kg | = | 500 ml |
| 20 ml/Kg | x 13.18 Kg | = | 263.6 ml |
| | | | 1763.6 ml divided by 2 = **881.8 ml** |

    b.    At what infusion rate?
          ml/hr = 881.8 ml/24 hr = **36.74 ml/hr**

73. Calculate the $M^2$ for a patient 73 cm tall who weighs 25.4 Kg.

$M^2 = \sqrt{73 \times 25.4/3600} = \sqrt{0.51506} = $ **0.72 $M^2$**

74. For the child whose $M^2$ you just calculated, for a medication ordered at 500 mg/$M^2$ per day in four divided doses, how much would the child receive per dose?

mg = 500 mg/$M^2$ x 0.72 $M^2$ = 360 mg/day x 1 day/4 doses = **90 mg/dose**
          per day

75. The usual dose of a medication, according to the literature, is 80-125 mg/Kg/day in three divided doses.

    a.    What is the safe range for your 82-lb patient?

mg    =    80 mg/Kg x 1 Kg/2.2 lb  x    82 lb  =    **2981.82 mg/day**
per day    **to**
125 mg/Kg x 1 Kg/2.2 lb  x    82 lb  =    **4659.09 mg/day**

Per dose range, dividing these by 3 doses is **993.94 – 1553.03 mg/dose**

    b.    The doctor has ordered 1 g of the medication every 6 hours. Is his order safe?

**Although he has ordered 4 times per day instead of 3, his order still falls within our calculated range both per dose and per day. It is therefore safe.**

76. Calculate the $M^2$ for a patient who weighs 54.16 lb and is 42.5 inches tall.

$\sqrt{24.62 \times 107.95 / 3600} = \sqrt{0.73826} =$ **0.86 $M^2$**

77. The doctor has ordered another medication for your patient in problem 76. His order reads "Give 400 mg/$M^2$." What will your patient's dose be?

mg = 400 mg/$M^2$ x 0.86 $M^2$ = **344 mg**

78. The doctor ordered maintenance fluids for your 107 lb patient. How much fluid will the patient receive in the next 24 hours, and at what rate will it infuse? Kg = 1 Kg/2.2 lb x 107 lb = 48.64 Kg

| | | | | |
|---|---|---|---|---|
| 100 ml/Kg | x | 10 Kg | = | 1000 ml |
| 50 ml/Kg | x | 10 Kg | = | 500 ml |
| 20 ml/Kg | x | 28.64 Kg | = | 572.8 ml |
| | | | | **2072.8 ml** |

ml/hr = 2072.8 ml/24 hr = **86.37 ml/hr**

79. Calculate the M² for an adolescent patient who is 5 ft 7 in tall and weighs 163 lb.

    cm = 2.54 cm/in x 67 in = 170.18 cm  Kg = 1 Kg/2.2 lb x 163 lb = 74.09 Kg

    M² = √ 170.18 x 74.09/3600 = √ 3.50240 = **1.87 M²**

80. The literature states the safe range for a medication is 30-50 mg/Kg/day in divided doses. The doctor has ordered 500 mg every 8 hours. The patient weighs 82 lb, and the medication comes in a 200 mg/5 ml concentration.

    a.  What is the safe range?

    30 mg/Kg x 37.27 Kg =  **1118.1 mg/day**  x 1 day/3 doses =  **372.7 mg/dose**
    Per day                             to                                          to
    50 g/Kg x 37.27 Kg =   **1863.5 mg/day** x 1 day/3 doses =  **621.17 mg/dose**

    b.  Is the doctor's order safe?
        **Yes**, it is within the calculated range, both per dose and per day.

    c.  How much will the child receive per dose, in ml?
        ml/dose = 5 ml/200 mg x 500 mg/dose = **12.5 ml/dose**

81. The child is to get a 350 ml bolus of D5 1/2 NS over the next 5 hours. What will the hourly rate be?

    ml/hr = 350 ml/5 hours = **70 ml/hr**

82. Calculate the safe dose for a medication ordered at 80 mg per M² for your patient, whose M² is 0.29.

    mg = 80 mg/M² x 0.29 M² = **23.2 mg**

83. Your patient weighs 6.4 Kg and is 33 cm long. The order is for him to receive 0.38 mg/Kg/day, or 10 mg per $M^2$, with the dose not to exceed 2.5 mg per day. Calculate the daily dose both ways, based on the doctor's order.

    $M^2 = \sqrt{6.4 \times 33}/3600 = \sqrt{0.05867} = 0.24\ M^2$   $10\ mg/M^2 \times 0.24\ M^2 = $ **2.4 mg**

    $0.38\ mg/Kg \times 6.4\ Kg = $ **2.43 mg**

84. Calculate the $M^2$ for a child who weighs 22 lb 9 oz and is 20 inches long.

    22 lb 9 oz = 22.5625 lb   Kg = 1 Kg/2.2 lb $\times$ 22.5625 lb = 10.26 Kg; cm = 2.54 cm/1 in $\times$ 20 in = 50.8 cm

    $M^2 = \sqrt{50.8 \times 10.26}/3600 = \sqrt{0.14478} = $ **0.38 $M^2$**

85. The doctor ordered 75 mg/$M^2$ three times daily for the child in the previous problem. How much medication will the child receive in one day?

    mg = 75 mg/$M^2$ $\times$ 0.38 $M^2$ = 28.5 mg/dose $\times$ 3 doses/day = **85.5 mg**

86. The child weighs 19.8 Kg, and the doctor orders 2 x maintenance fluids to be infused over the next 24 hours. At what rate will you set the pump?

    | | | |
    |---|---|---|
    | 100 ml/Kg x 10 Kg | = | 1000 ml |
    | 50 ml/Kg x 9.8 Kg | = | 490 ml |
    | | | 1490 ml x 2 = 2980 ml |

    ml/hr = 2980 ml/24 hours = **124.17 ml/hr**

87. Your patient has an NG tube, through which she has lost 173 ml in the past 12 hours. The doctor has ordered D5W with 10 mEq of KCl as replacement fluids. The patient currently has D5NS infusing. What rate will you set on the pump to infuse the NG replacement fluid?

    ml/hr = 173 ml/12 hours = **14.42 ml/hr**

88. The safe range for the ordered medication is 25 to 50 mg/Kg/day in divided doses. The doctor has ordered 100 mg every 6 hours for your 18.7 Kg patient. Is his order safe?

   25 mg/Kg x 18.7 Kg = 467.5 mg/day (116.88 mg/dose); 50 mg/Kg x 18.7 Kg = 935 Kg/day (233.75 mg/dose)

   MD ordered 100 mg/dose x 4 doses = 400 mg/day, so both per dose and per day it is **not safe.** Both fall below the safe ranges we have calculated.

89. Your patient weighs 11.4 Kg. The literature states the usual dose of a medication is 20 mg/Kg. What is the safe dose for the medication?

   20 mg/Kg x 11.4 Kg = **228 mg**

90. Calculate the $M^2$ of a patient who is 117 cm tall and weighs 28.18 Kg.

   $M^2 = \sqrt{117 \times 28.18 / 3600} = \sqrt{0.91585} = \textbf{0.96 } \mathbf{M^2}$

91. For the child in the previous problem, what is the dosage range for a drug with a recommended dose of 5 to 15 mg/$M^2$?

   mg = 5 mg/$M^2$ x 0.96 $M^2$ =    **4.8 mg**
                                        **to**
   mg = 15 mg/$M^2$ x 0.96 $M^2$ =   **14.4 mg**

92. The doctor has ordered a medication at 150 mg/$M^2$, or 10 mg/Kg/dose. Calculate your patient's dose both ways. The child's $M^2$ is 1.33, and she weighs 20 Kg.

   mg = 150 mg/$M^2$ x 1.33 $M^2$ = **199.5 mg**
   mg = 10 mg/Kg x 20 Kg = **200 mg**

93. The doctor has ordered a medication at 500 mg every 6 hours. Your reference states the safe dosage is 60 – 100 mg/Kg/day in divided doses. Your patient weighs 31.2 Kg. The medication is available in an oral form with a concentration of 25 mg/ml.

   a.   Is the doctor's order safe?

   60 mg/Kg x 31.2 Kg = 1872 mg/day x 1 day/4 doses = 468 mg/dose
     per day                      to                               to
   100 mg/Kg x 31.2 Kg = 3120 mg/day x 1 day/4 doses = 780 mg/dose
   **The doctor's order is safe, both per dose and per day.**

   b.   How much will the child get per day, in ml?

   ml = 1 ml/25 mg x 500 mg/6 hr x 24 hr/1 day = **80 ml/day**

94. The patient has NS infusing at 25 ml/hr. He has an NG tube, through which he has lost 200 ml during the shift prior to yours. The doctor has ordered replacement fluids of D5NS. At what rate should the replacement fluids infuse?

   ml/hr = 200 ml/12 hours = **16.67 ml/hr** of D5NS
   NS will continue to infuse at 25 ml/hr on a separate pump.

95. The order is for a medication at 150 mg/$M^2$ for your patient, who has an $M^2$ of 0.57. How much should you give your patient, per the doctor's order?

   mg = 150 mg/$M^2$ x 0.57 $M^2$ = **85.5 mg**

96. The safe range for the medication in the previous problem is 1.5 to 3.25 mg/Kg/day. Your patient weighs 25 Kg.

   a.   What is the safe range for your patient?
   1.5 mg/Kg x 25 Kg = **37.5 mg**
       per day                **to**        per day
   3.25 mg/Kg x 25 Kg = **81.25 mg**

   b.   Based on this, was the doctor's order in problem 95 safe?
   **No. The doctor's order of 85.5 mg exceeds the safe range.**

97. The order is for 1.5 x maintenance fluids for your patient, who weighs 21.7 Kg. How much fluid will you give your patient in the next 24 hours, in compliance with the order?

| 100 ml/Kg x 10 Kg | = | 1000 ml |
|---|---|---|
| 50 ml/Kg x 10 Kg | = | 500 ml |
| 20 ml/Kg x 1.7 Kg | = | 34 ml |

1534 ml x 1.5 = **2301 ml**

98. The patient has lost 258 ml via NG tube in the previous shift. IV fluids infusing are D5 1/2 NS at 45 ml/hr. Replacement fluids are D5 1/2 NS. At what rate will you set the pump to return the fluid lost to the NG over the next 12 hours?

258ml/12 hr = 21.5 ml/hr + 45 ml/hr = **66.5 ml/hr**
Ordered fluids are the same, can run at the same time through the same pump.

99. The literature states the safe range of a medication is 75 – 125 mg/Kg/day in four divided doses. Your patient weighs 59 Kg. What is the safe per dose range for her?

75 mg/Kg x 59 Kg = 4425 mg/day x 1 day/4 doses = **1106.25 mg/dose**
　　Per day　　　　　　　　to　　　　　　　　　　　　**to**
125 mg/Kg x 59 Kg = 7375 mg/day x 1 day/4 doses = **1843.75 mg/dose**

100. Your patient weighs 13 lb 7 oz. The MD has ordered a medication at 28 mcg/Kg/min. The medication is available 150 mg in 100 ml. At what rate will you set the pump?

13 lb 7 oz = 6.11 Kg

ml/hr = 100 ml/150 mg x 1 mg/1000 mcg x  28 mcg/Kg  x 6.11 Kg = 0.11405 ml/min x 60 min/1 hr = **6.84 ml/hr**
　　　　　　　　　　　　　　　　　　　　　per min

101. Your pediatric patient weighs 15.8 Kg. The antibiotic ordered has a concentration of 500 mg/20ml. The usual dose is 20 to 40 mg/Kg/day in three divided doses.

a. The doctor has ordered 300 mg/dose. Is this a safe dose?
mg = 20 mg/Kg x 15.8 Kg = 316 mg/day = 105.33 mg/dose
    per day
mg = 40 mg/Kg x 15.8 Kg = 632 mg/day = 210.67 mg/dose

**The dose is unsafe.**

b. The doctor changed the order to 100 mg/dose. Is this an accurate dose?
**No.** It is below the bottom of the per dose safe range, so is **unsafe.**

c. The doctor changes the order again, to 225 mg/dose. Is this dose accurate and safe?
**No.** The dose is now above the top of the per dose safe range, so is **unsafe.**

102. The child weighs 47 pounds, and has a moderately severe infection. Kefzol has been ordered. For a moderately severe infection, Kefzol is to be given at 25 to 50 mg/Kg/day.

a. What is the safe range for this medication?
mg = 25 mg/Kg x 1 Kg/2.2 lb x 47 lb = **534.09 mg/day**
    per day
mg = 50 mg/Kg x 1 Kg/2.2 lb x 47 lb = **1068.18 mg/day**

b. If the medication is given in 4 divided doses, what will the per dose range be?

Per dose is     534.09 mg/day x 1 day/4 doses = **133.52 mg**
                  1068.18 mg/day x 1 day/4 doses = **267.05 mg**

c. The doctor has ordered 150 mg every 6 hours. Should you question the order?

**There is no reason to question the order.** It is safe, both per dose and per day.

103. Dopamine comes in 5 ml vials with a concentration of 200 mg/5 ml. The doctor's order is for "Dopamine 3 mcg/Kg/min IV. Dilute 100 mg dopamine in 100 ml D5 1/2 NS." The child weighs 16 pounds.

    a.    How many ml dopamine should be added to the 100 ml D5 1/2 NS to reach the ordered dilution?

        ml = 5 ml/200 mg x 100 mg = **2.5 ml**

    b.    How many mcg should the child receive per hour?

        mcg/hr = 3 mcg/Kg x 1 Kg/2.2 lb x 16 lb = 21.82 mcg/min x 60 min/hr = **1309.2 mcg/hr** per min.

    c.    What would the flow rate be to infuse this dose?

        ml/hr = 102.5 ml/100 mg x 1 mg/1000 mcg x 1309.2 mcg/hr = **1.34 ml/hr**

104. Calculate the BSA ($M^2$) of a teenager who weighs 47.81 Kg and is 161.3 cm tall.

    $M^2 = \sqrt{47.81 \times 161.3/3600} = \sqrt{2.14215} =$ **1.46 $M^2$**

105. The recommended child's dose is 5 to 10 mg/$M^2$. Based on the $M^2$ you just calculated in problem 104, what is the recommended dose range for this teenager?

    mg = 5 mg/$M^2$ x 1.46 $M^2$ = **7.3 mg**
    mg = 10 mg/$M^2$ x 1.46 $M^2$ = **14.6 mg**

106. A cancer drug is ordered for a patient whose BSA is 1.31 $M^2$. The doctor orders 25 mg/$M^2$ IV. What dose will your patient receive?

    mg = 25 mg/$M^2$ x 1.31 $M^2$ = **32.75 mg**

107. A child weighing 17.63 Kg has an antibiotic ordered at 500 mg every 6 hours. The child's dosage in your reference for this medication is 80 – 200 mg/Kg/day in divided doses. The drug is available in a 250 mg/ml concentration.

    a.    How many mg will the child receive per day?
        mg = 500 mg/6 hr x 24 hr = **2000 mg**

    b.    Is the drug dosage ordered per day within safe parameters?
        mg = 80 mg/Kg x 17.63 Kg = 1410.4 mg/day = 352.6 mg/dose
            per day
        mg = 200 mg/Kg x 17.63 Kg = 3526 mg/day = 881.5 mg/dose

**Yes, the order is safe.**

    c.    How many ml will the child receive per dose?
        ml = 1 ml/250 mg x 500 mg = **2 ml**

108. Your patient weighs 18.62 Kg. The doctor has ordered the patient to receive 14 mg/hr of a medication which comes in a concentration of 2.8 mg/ml.

    a.    How many mcg/min/Kg will the patient receive?

        mcg/min = 1000 mcg/1 mg x 14 mg/60 min = 233.33 mcg/min
        233.33 mcg/min divided by 18.62 Kg = **12.53 mcg/min/Kg**

    b.    At what rate will you set the pump to deliver this medication?

        ml/hr = 1 ml/2.8 mg x 1 mg/1000 mcg x 233.33 mcg/min x 60 min/hr = **5 ml/hr**

109. The doctor has ordered 1.5 x maintenance fluids for your pediatric patient, who weighs 24.77 Kg. How much fluid will your patient receive in the next 24 hours?

    100 ml/Kg x 10 Kg   =    1000 ml
    50 ml/Kg x 10 Kg    =    500 ml
    20 ml/Kg x 4.77 Kg  =    95.4 ml
                           1595.4 ml x 1.5 = **2393.1 ml**

110. The doctor orders a medication at 3.5 mg/Kg/day, in three divided doses. Your patient weighs 36 pounds. The medication comes in 10 ml vials containing 100 mg of medication.

    a.    How many mg will the child receive per dose?

        mg = 3.5 mg/Kg x 1 Kg/2.2 lb x 36 lb = 57.27 mg/day = **19.09 mg/dose**
            per day

    b.    Per day?

        As shown in the work for part (a), **57.27 mg/day.**

    c.    How many ml per dose?

        ml = 10 ml/100 mg x 19.09 mg = **1.91 ml**

111. The order is for erythromycin 125 mg every 4 hours. The child weighs 29 lb. The desired range for this antibiotic is 30 – 50 mg/Kg/day in divided doses. The available medication comes 125 mg/5 ml.

    a.    Is the ordered dose safe?

        mg = 30 mg/Kg x 1 Kg/2.2 lb x 29 lb = 395.45 mg/day = 65.91 mg/dose
            per day
        mg = 50 mg/Kg x 1 Kg/2.2 lb x 29 lb = 659.09 mg/day = 109.85 mg/dose
        **The order is unsafe**, too high both per dose and per day.

    b.    How many ml will the child receive per dose, per the MD's order?

        ml = 5 ml/125 mg x 125 mg = **5 ml**

112. The doctor has ordered 80 mg of a medication every 8 hours. The child weighs 18.9 lb. Referenced dosage is 30 mg/Kg/day in divided doses. The medication is available in a concentration of 150 mg/5 ml.

    a.    Is the prescribed dose safe?
        mg = 30 mg/Kg x 1 Kg/2.2 lb x 18.9 lb = 257.73 mg/day = 85.91 mg/dose
        **The order is unsafe**, falling below the safe dose both per dose and per day.

    b.    How many ml should the child receive per dose, by the MD's order?
ml = 5 ml/150 mg x 80 mg = **2.67 ml**

113.    The order is for digoxin 30 mcg every 12 hours. Your patient weighs 9.74 Kg. Your reference states a safe dosage is 0.006 – 0.012 mg/Kg/day. Available is digoxin 50 mcg/ml.

    a.    Is the prescribed dose safe?
mcg = 6 mcg/Kg x 9.74 Kg = 58.44 mcg/day = 29.22 mcg/dose
      per day
mcg = 12 mcg/Kg x 9.74 Kg = 116.88 mcg/day = 58.44 mcg/dose

**The order is safe, both per dose and per day.**

    b.    How many ml a dose will the child receive, per the MD's order?
ml = 1 ml/50 mcg x 30 mcg = **0.6 ml**

114.    Your pediatric patient weighs 18.92 lb. The medication ordered has a concentration of 300 mg to 15 ml. The usual dose is 10 – 15 mg/Kg/day in two divided doses.

    a.    The doctor ordered 150 mg a day, divided into two doses. Is this a safe dose?
mg = 10 mg/Kg x 1 Kg/2.2 lb x 18.92 lb = 86 mg/day = 43 mg/dose
      per day
mg = 15 mg/Kg x 1 Kg/2.2 lb x 18.92 lb = 129 mg/day = 64.5 mg/dose
**No, the order is too high, both per dose and per day, so is unsafe.**

    b.    The doctor changed the order to 30 mg a dose with three doses a day. Is this safe?
**No.** This is 90 mg/day, so it falls within the safe per day range. However, 30 mg/dose is below the safe per dose range of 43 – 64.5/dose. If <u>either</u> per day <u>or</u> per dose is unsafe, the order is considered **unsafe.**

    c.    How much would you give in ml per dose for the doctor's 2nd order?
ml = 15 ml/300 mg x 30 mg = **1.5 ml**

115.    The doctor has ordered an antibiotic for your 24-lb. pediatric patient. The antibiotic is to be given at 20 – 40 mg/Kg/day.

    a.    What is the safe range for this antibiotic?
mg = 20 mg/Kg x 1 Kg/2.2 lb x 24 lb = **218.18 mg/day**
      per day
mg = 40 mg/Kg x 1 Kg/2.2 lb x 24 lb = **436.36 mg/day**

b.   If the child is to get three doses per day, what is the per dose range?
     mg = 218.18 mg/3 doses = **72.73 mg /dose**
     mg = 436.36 mg/3 doses = **145.45 mg/dose**

116.  Calculate the M² for a teenaged patient who is 5'2" tall and weighs 127 lb.

     cm = 2.54 cm/in x 62 in = 157.48 cm   Kg = 1 Kg/2.2 lb x 127 lb = 57.73 Kg
     M² = √157.48 x 57.73/3600 = √2.52537 = **1.59 M²**

117.  A medication has been ordered for a child which is to be given at 15 mg/M². Using the M² you just calculated in problem 116, what dose will the child receive?

     mg = 15 mg/M² x 1.59 M² = **23.85 mg**

118.  The doctor ordered half maintenance fluids on your 34.52 Kg patient. What rate will you set on the pump to infuse these fluids in 12 hours?

     100 ml/Kg x 10 Kg    =      1000 ml
     50 ml/Kg x 10 Kg     =      500 ml
     20 ml/Kg x 14.52 Kg =       290.4 ml
                                 1790.4 ml/2 = 895.2 ml

     ml/hr = 895.2ml/12 hr = **74.6 ml/hr**

119.  Your pediatric patient has had abdominal surgery and now has an NG tube, which has suctioned 70 ml out in the past 12 hours. He has D5 1/2 NS with 20 mEq KCl infusing at 40 ml/hr. The doctor has ordered D5 1/2 NS with 20 mEq KCl for replacement of fluids lost via NG. To what rate should you reset the IV flow rate to follow the doctor's order?

     ml/hr = 70 ml/12 hr =      5.83 ml/hr
                                +40 ml/hr
                                **45.83 ml/hr**

     Because the fluids are identical, they can infuse together. At the end of the 12 hours, the flow rate will be reset to its original 40 ml/hr (unless, of course, there are again replacement fluids to infuse).

120. A child who weighs 83 lb. is to receive a medication which has been ordered at 1 g every 8 hours. Your reference states that a child's safe dose for the medication is 75 to 125 mg/Kg/day in divided doses. The drug comes in a 100 mg/ml concentration.

   a.   How much (in mg) will the child receive per day, by the MD's order?
        mg = 1000 mg/dose x 3 doses = **3000 mg**

   b.   Is the doctor's order safe?
        mg = 75 mg/Kg x 1 Kg/2.2 lb x 83 lb = 2829.55 mg/day = 943.18 mg/dose
              per day
        mg = 125 mg/Kg x 1 Kg/2.2 lb x 83 lb = 4715.91 mg/day = 1571.97 mg/dose
        **The order is safe.**

   c.   How many ml will the child receive per dose?
        ml = 1 ml/100 mg x 1000 mg/dose = **10 ml**

121. Calculate the $M^2$ for a child who weighs 14.75 Kg and is 43.6 cm tall.

   $M^2 = \sqrt{14.75 \times 43.6/3600} = \sqrt{0.17864} =$ **0.42 $M^2$**

122. The child is to receive 5 – 10 mg/$M^2$. Using the $M^2$ calculated in problem 121, what is the child's safe range of medication?

   mg = 5 mg/$M^2$ x 0.42 $M^2$ = **2.1 mg**
   mg = 10 mg/$M^2$ x 0.42 $M^2$ = **4.2 mg**

123. The doctor has ordered a medication at 7 mg/Kg/day in four divided doses. The patient weighs 44 lb. Your reference states the safe range is 30 – 40 mg every 8 hours.

   a.   How much will the child receive per dose under the doctor's order?
        mg = 7 mg/Kg x 1 Kg/2.2 lb x 44 lb = 140 mg/day = **35 mg/dose**
              per day

   b.   Is the doctor's order safe?
        mg = 30 mg/dose x 3 doses = 90 mg/day
        mg = 40 mg/dose x 3 doses = 120 mg/day

   **The order is unsafe.** Although his 35 mg/dose falls within the safe per dose range of 30 – 40 mg, because he has ordered 4 doses a day, his daily total is 140 mg, above the 120 mg top of the safe per day range.

124. The medication is infusing at 23 ml/hr on a pump. The medicine is available 10 mg in 100 ml D5W. How many mcg/min/Kg is the patient receiving, for a 14.54 Kg patient?

mcg/min   =   1000 mcg/mg x 10 mg/100 ml x 23 ml/60 min = 38.33 mcg/min
38.33 mcg/min divided by 14.54 Kg = **2.64 mcg/min/Kg**

125. The doctor has ordered IV fluids of D5 1/2 NS at 40 ml/hr for your post-op pediatric patient. The patient has an NG tube, which has drained 105 ml on the previous shift. NG replacement fluids ordered are D5NS with 20 mEq KCl. Determine how much you would give, and how you would set the pump or pumps.

**Pump #1** IV fluids **40 ml/hr** will continue to infuse, as before

**Pump #2** replacement fluids 105ml/12 hr = **8.75 ml/hr**

126. A medication has been ordered 60 mcg/Kg/min for your pediatric patient. The medication comes in 25 ml vials containing 1 g of the medication. It is to be mixed to create a solution of 1000 mg in a 500 ml bag. The child weighs 30 Kg.

    a. How many ml of the medication should be added to the 500 ml bag to get the ordered strength?
    ml = 25 ml/1000 mg x 1000 mg = **25 ml**

    b. How many mg of the medication should the child receive per hour?
    mg/hr = 1 mg/1000 mcg x 60 mcg/Kg x 30 Kg = 1.8 mg/min x 60 min/hr = **108 mg/hr**
                                    per min

    c. What flow rate should be set to infuse the medication per the doctor's order?
    ml/hr = 525 ml/1000 mg x 108 mg/hr = **56.7 ml/hr**

127. Your teen-aged patient has ovarian cancer. The initial round of the medication ordered is to be given at 260 mg/M$^2$/day in four divided doses for 21 days. The medication comes in 50 mg capsules. Your patient weighs 118 lb. and is 63 in. tall. How much should she receive per dose? How many capsules will this be per dose?

cm = 2.54 cm/in x 63 in = 160.02 cm    Kg = 1 Kg/2.2 lb = 53.64 Kg
M$^2$ = $\sqrt{53.64 \times 160.02/3600}$ = $\sqrt{2.3843}$ = 1.54 M$^2$
mg = 260 mg/M$^2$ x 1.54 M$^2$ = 400.4 mg/day = **100.1 mg/dose**
        per day
cap = 1 cap/50 mg x 100.1 mg/dose = **2 caps**

128. A medication is ordered at 70 mg every 6 hours for a 17 lb. 9 oz. child. The literature states safe dosage is 30 mg/Kg/day. The available medication: 500 mg in 250 ml of 0.45 NS.

    a.    What is the child's weight in Kg?
        Kg = 1 Kg/2.2 lb x 17.5625 lb = **7.98 Kg**

    b.    How many mg/day will the child receive by the doctor's order?
        mg = 70 mg/dose x 4 doses/day = **280 mg/day**

    c.    Is the doctor's order safe, by the literature?
        mg = 30 mg/Kg x 7.98 Kg = 239.4 mg/day = 59.85 mg/dose per day
        **Unsafe**, per dose and per day

    d.    What will be the ml per dose, by the doctor's order?
        ml = 250 ml/500 mg x 70 mg = **35 ml**

129. A 54-pound child has an order for 250 mg of an antibiotic four times daily. The antibiotic come at 100 mg/5 ml, with the usual dose 15 – 40 mg/Kg/day in three divided doses.

    mg = 15 mg/Kg x 1 Kg/2.2 lb x 54 lb = 368.18 mg/day = **122.73 mg/dose** per day
    mg = 40 mg/Kg x 1 Kg/2.2 lb x 54 lb = 981.82 mg/day = **327.27 mg/dose**

    b.    Is the doctor's order safe?
        **No**. He has ordered 250 mg/dose x 4 doses/day = 1000 mg/day, above the top of the safe per day range.

    c.    How many ml should the child receive per dose, following the MD's order?
        ml = 5 ml/100 mg x 250 mg = **12.5 ml**

130. Your fragile 13-month-old HIV-positive patient has developed a herpes simplex infection. The doctor has ordered acyclovir sodium 30 mg/Kg/day in three divided doses. The child weighs 26 pounds and is 28 inches long.

    a.    What is her $M^2$?
        cm = 2.54 cm/in x 28 in = 71.12 cm    Kg = 1 Kg/2.2 lb x 26 lb = 11.82 Kg
        $M^2 = \sqrt{71.12 \times 11.82/3600} = \sqrt{0.23351} =$ **0.48 $M^2$**

b.  The label reads 750 mg/M² per day for 7 days. What is the per dose and per day safe dose for this child?

mg = 750 mg/M² x 0.48 M² = **360 mg/day** = **120 mg/dose**

c.  Is the doctor's order safe?

mg = 30 mg/Kg/day x 11.82 Kg = 354.6 mg/day = 118.2 mg/dose

Strictly by the rules, the doctor's order is <u>not</u> safe, as it is not exactly according to the literature. However, both per day and per dose, he is at 98.5% of the accurate dose per literature. The facility may well have a policy which allows the dose to be given. However, the nurse would need to make the calls necessary to be sure before administering the dose.

131.  Your patient weighs 17 Kg and is 82 cm tall. What is his M²?

$$M^2 = \sqrt{17 \times 82/3600} = \sqrt{0.38722} = \mathbf{0.62\ M^2}$$

132.  Your patient is to receive 2 – 5 mg/M² of a medication. Based on the M² you calculated in the previous problem, what is the safe dose range?

mg = 2 mg/M² x 0.62 M² = **1.24 mg**
mg = 5 mg/M² x 0.62 M² = **3.1 mg**

133.  A child weighing 8 lb 7 oz is to receive a medication at 6 mcg/Kg/min. The medication is available 100 mg in 100 ml. At what rate would you set a pump to infuse the correct amount?

Kg = 1 Kg/2.2 lb x 8.4375 lb = 3.84 Kg

ml/hr = 100 ml/100 mg x 1 mg/1000 mcg x 6 mcg/Kg x 3.84 Kg = 0.023 ml/min
per min

0.023 ml/min x 60 min/hr = **1.38 ml/hr**

134. The child weighs 44 lb. The medication's safe dose is 15 to 25 mg/Kg/day in four divided doses. The doctor has ordered 100 mg/dose. Is his order safe?

mg = 15 mg/Kg x 1 Kg/2.2 lb x 44 lb = 300 mg/day = 75 mg/dose
    per day
mg = 25 mg/Kg x 1 Kg/2.2 lb x 44 lb = 500 mg/day = 125 mg/dose

**The order is safe.**

135. A child has been admitted. The child is 3'8" tall and weighs 55 lb. Her medication has been ordered at 14 mg/M² per dose. How much will you give per dose?

cm = 2.54 cm/in x 44 in = 111.76 cm; Kg = 1 Kg/2.2 lb x 55 lb = 25 Kg
$M^2 = \sqrt{111.76 \times 25}/3600 = \sqrt{0.77611} = 0.88\ M^2$
mg = 14 mg/M² x 0.88 M² = **12.32 mg**

136. The child has an NG tube which has drained 135 ml in the past 12 hours. IV fluids are ½ NS at 40 ml/hr. Replacement fluids ordered are ½ NS with 20 mEq potassium. At what rate will you set the pump to replace the fluid lost to the NG tube?

ml/hr = 135 ml/12 hr = **11.25 ml/hr**

137. Your pediatric patient has an antibiotic ordered which is available at 300 mg/10 ml in a suspension. The patient weighs 16.9 Kg. The usual order is 20 – 30 mg/Kg/day in three divided doses. The doctor has ordered 250 mg/dose. Is this dose safe?

**The order is unsafe.**

mg = 20 mg/Kg x 16.9 Kg = 338 mg/day = 112.67 mg/dose
    per day
mg = 30 mg/Kg x 16.9 Kg = 507 mg/day = 169 mg/dose

## Questions 138 – 140 are related

138. The medication is available in a concentration of 100 mg/5 ml in 10 ml vials. The directions indicate you are to dilute 30 mg of the medication in 50 ml of D5W. How much of the medication should be added to the 50 ml of D5W to get the desired dilution?

ml = 5 ml/100 mg x 30 mg = **1.5 ml**

139. Your 15.4 Kg patient is to receive 8 mcg/Kg/min of the above medication. How much will they receive per hour?

mcg/hr = 8 mcg/Kg x 15.4 Kg = 123.2 mcg/min x 60 min/hr = **7392 mcg/hr**
 per min

140. What flow rate would you set to infuse this dose?

ml/hr = 51.5 ml/30 mg x 1 mg/1000 mcg x 7392 mcg/hr = **12.69 ml/hr**

141. The doctor has ordered 70 mg of a medication every 12 hours. The child weighs 11 lb 5 oz. The drug dosage for the medication in the literature is 25 mg/Kg/day in divided doses. Is the dose the doctor ordered safe?

mg = 25 mg/Kg x 1 Kg/2.2 lb x 11.3125 lb = 128.55 mg/day = 64.28 mg/dose
 per day
**The order is unsafe**, both per dose and per day.

142. What is the $M^2$ of a patient weighing 48.7 Kg who is 142.8 cm tall?

$M^2 = \sqrt{48.7 \times 142.8/3600} = \sqrt{1.93177} = $ **1.39 $M^2$**

143. The doctor has ordered 1.5 x maintenance fluids for your 29.54 Kg patient. At what rate will you set the pump to infuse these fluids over the next 24 hours?

     100 ml/Kg x 10 Kg    =    1000 ml
     50 ml/Kg x 10 Kg     =    500 ml
     20 ml/Kg x 9.54 Kg   =    190.8 ml
                               1690.8 ml x 1.5 = 2536.2 ml

     ml/hr = 2536.2 ml/24 hours = **105.68 ml/hr**

144. The child has ½ maintenance fluids ordered. He weighs 11.1 Kg. How much should he get in the next 24 hours? What flow rate would you set to deliver this?

     100 ml/Kg x 10 Kg    =    1000 ml
     50 ml/Kg x 1.1 Kg    =    55 ml
                               1055 ml/2 = 527.5 ml

     ml/hr = 527.5 ml/24 hours = **21.98 ml/hr**

145. What is the M² of a patient who is 4'7" tall and weighs 68 lb?

     cm = 2.54 cm/in x 55 in = 139.7 cm; Kg = 1 Kg/2.2 lb x 68 lb = 30.91 Kg

     $M^2 = \sqrt{139.7 \times 30.91/3600} = \sqrt{1.19948} =$ **1.1 M²**

146. The doctor has ordered a 500 ml bolus dose of D5 1/2 NS for your pediatric patient, who currently has D5 1/2 NS infusing at 35 ml/hr. At what rate will you set the pump to infuse the bolus dose over the next four hours?

     ml/hr = 500 ml/4 hr = 125 ml/hr but the fluids are the same, so
     ml/hr = 125 ml/hr + 35 ml/hr = **160 ml/hr**

147. Your patient is 50 inches tall. She weighs 78 lb. She is to receive 24 mg/M² per dose of an ordered medication. How much will you give?

cm = 2.54 cm/in x 50 in = 127 cm; Kg = 1 Kg/2.2 lb x 78 lb = 35.45 Kg
M² = √127 x 35.45/3600 = √1.2506 = 1.12 M²
mg = 24 mg/M² x 1.12 M² = **26.88 mg**

148. The five-year-old patient, who weighs 52 lb, has a severe ear infection, and the doctor has prescribed amoxicillin in a liquid form with a concentration of 125 mg in 5 ml. The usual dose is 20 – 40 mg/Kg/day in three divided doses. The doctor has ordered 300 mg every 6 hours.

   a.   What is the safe range?
   mg =20 mg/Kg x 1 Kg/2.2 lb x 52 lb = 472.73 mg/day = **157.58 mg/dose**
           per day
   mg = 40 mg/Kg x 1 Kg/2.2 lb x 52 lb = 945.45 mg/day = **315.15 mg/dose**

   b.   Is the doctor's order safe?
   **No.** It is within the safe per dose range, but he has ordered 4 doses a day, which is 1200 mg. This exceeds the safe per day range. If any part is unsafe, the order is unsafe.

149. The 8-year-old post-op patient has received an accidental narcotic overdose, and is now unresponsive. The doctor orders 0.5 ml Narcan to counteract the narcotic. The child weighs 66 pounds. Safe dose is 0.005 to 0.01 mg/Kg, and the Narcan is available 400 mcg/ml. What is the safe range, and is the doctor's order safe?

mg = 0.005 mg/Kg x 1 Kg/2.2 lb x 66 lb = **0.15 mg**
mg = 0.01 mg/Kg x 1 Kg/2.2 lb x 66 lb = **0.3 mg**

Doctor's order is 1 mg/1000 mcg x 400 mcg/ml x 0.5 ml = 0.2 mg so the **order is safe.**

150. Your pediatric cancer patient is to receive doxorubicin 30 mg a week. The child is 42 inches tall and weighs 57 lb. The medication is available 25 mg in 50 ml of D5W. Safe dose is 20 – 30 mg/M² once a week.

   a.   What is the child's M²?
   cm = 2.54 cm/in x 42 in = 106.68 cm; Kg = 1 Kg/2.2 lb x 57 lb = 25.91 Kg
   M² = √106.68 x 25.91/3600 = √0.7678 = **0.88 M²**

b. What is the safe range for the medication for this child?
   mg = 20 mg/M$^2$ x 0.88 M$^2$ = **17.6 mg per week**
   mg = 30 mg/M$^2$ x 0.88 M$^2$ = **26.4 mg per week**

c. Is the doctor's order safe?
   At 30 mg per week, the **order is unsafe.**

d. How many ml will the child receive per dose by the doctor's order?
   ml = 50 ml/25 mg x 30 mg = **60 ml**

Made in the USA
San Bernardino,
CA

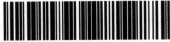